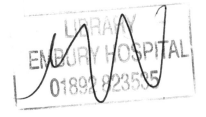

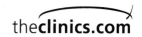

# OBSTETRICS AND GYNECOLOGY CLINICS

## OF NORTH AMERICA

### Diabetes in Pregnancy

GUEST EDITOR
Deborah L. Conway, MD

CONSULTING EDITOR
William F. Rayburn, MD

June 2007 • Volume 34 • Number 2

**SAUNDERS**

An Imprint of Elsevier, Inc.
PHILADELPHIA   LONDON   TORONTO   MONTREAL   SYDNEY   TOKYO

**W.B. SAUNDERS COMPANY**
*A Division of Elsevier Inc.*

Elsevier, Inc. • 1600 John F. Kennedy Blvd. • Suite 1800 • Philadelphia, PA 19103-2899

http://www.theclinics.com

**OBSTETRICS AND GYNECOLOGY**
**CLINICS OF NORTH AMERICA**
June 2007
Editor: Carla Holloway

Volume 34, Number 2
ISSN 0889-8545
ISBN 1-4160-4344-6
978-1-4160-4344-7

The ideas and opinions expressed in *Obstetrics and Gynecology Clinics of North America* do not necessarily reflect those of the Publisher. The Publisher does not assume any responsibility for any injury and/or damage to persons or property arising out of or related to any use of the material contained in this periodical. The reader is advised to check the appropriate medical literature and the product information currently provided by the manufacturer of each drug to be administered to verify the dosage, the method and duration of administration, or contraindications. It is the responsibility of the treating physician or other health care professional, relying on independent experience and knowledge of the patient, to determine drug dosages and the best treatment for the patient. Mention of any product in this issue should not be construed as endorsement by the contributors, editors, or the Publisher of the product or manufacturers' claims.

*Obstetrics and Gynecology Clinics* (ISSN 0889-8545) is published quarterly by Elsevier Inc., 360 Park Avenue South, New York, NY 10010-1710. Months of issue are March, June, September, and December. Business and Editorial Offices: 1600 John F. Kennedy Blvd., Suite 1800, Philadelphia, PA 19103-2899. Customer Service Office: 6277 Sea Harbor Drive, Orlando, FL 32887-4800. Periodicals postage paid at New York, NY, and additional mailing offices. Subscription prices are $407.00 per year Institutional, $330.00 per year Institutional USA, $407.00 per year Institutional Canada, $265.00 per year Personal, $194.00 per year Personal USA, $232.00 per year Personal Canada, $135.00 per year Personal student, $97.00 per year Personal student USA, $135.00 per year Personal student Canada. To receive student/resident rate, orders must be accompanied by name of affiliated institution, date of term, and the signature of program/residency coordinator on institution letterhead. Orders will be billed at individual rate until proof of status is received. Foreign air speed delivery is included in all Clinics subscription prices. All prices are subject to change without notice. POSTMASTER: Send address changes to *Obstetrics and Gynecology Clinics*, Elsevier Periodicals Customer Service, 6277 Sea Harbor Drive, Orlando, FL 32887-4800. **Customer Service: 1-800-654-2452 (US). From outside of the US, call 1-407-345-4000.**

*Obstetrics and Gynecology Clinics of North America* is also published in Spanish by Mc Graw-Hill Interamericana Editores S.A., P.O. Box 5-237, 06500, Mexico; in Portuguese by Reichmann and Affonso Editores, Rio de Janeiro, Brazil; and in Greek by Paschalidis Medical Publications, Athens, Greece.

*Obstetrics and Gynecology Clinics of North America* is covered in *Index Medicus, Excerpta Medica, Current Concepts/Clinical Medicine, Science Citation Index, BIOSIS, CINAHL, and ISI/BIOMED.*

Printed in the United States of America.

## GOAL STATEMENT

The goal of *Obstetrics and Gynecology Clinics of North America* is to keep practicing physicians up to date with current clinical practice in OB/GYN by providing timely articles reviewing the state of the art in patient care.

## ACCREDITATION

The *Obstetrics and Gynecology Clinics of North America* is planned and implemented in accordance with the Essential Areas and Policies of the Accreditation Council for Continuing Medical Education (ACCME) through the joint sponsorship of the University of Virginia School of Medicine and Elsevier. The University of Virginia School of Medicine is accredited by the ACCME to provide continuing medical education for physicians.

The University of Virginia School of Medicine designates this educational activity for a maximum of 15 *AMA PRA Category 1 Credits™*. Physicians should only claim credit commensurate with the extent of their participation in the activity.

The American Medical Association has determined that physicians not licensed in the US who participate in this CME activity are eligible for *AMA PRA Category 1 Credits™*.

Category 1 credit can be earned by reading the text material, taking the CME examination online at *http:// www.theclinics.com/home/cme*, and completing the evaluation. After taking the test, you will be required to review any and all incorrect answers. Following completion of the test and evaluation, your credit will be awarded and you may print your certificate.

## FACULTY DISCLOSURE/CONFLICT OF INTEREST

The University of Virginia School of Medicine, as an ACCME accredited provider, endorses and strives to comply with the Accreditation Council for Continuing Medical Education (ACCME) Standards of Commercial Support, Commonwealth of Virginia statutes, University of Virginia policies and procedures, and associated federal and private regulations and guidelines on the need for disclosure and monitoring of proprietary and financial interests that may affect the scientific integrity and balance of content delivered in continuing medical education activities under our auspices.

The University of Virginia School of Medicine requires that all CME activities accredited through this institution be developed independently and be scientifically rigorous, balanced and objective in the presentation/discussion of its content, theories and practices.

All authors/editors participating in an accredited CME activity are expected to disclose to the readers relevant financial relationships with commercial entities occurring within the past 12 months (such as grants or research support, employee, consultant, stock holder, member of speakers bureau, etc.). The University of Virginia School of Medicine will employ appropriate mechanisms to resolve potential conflicts of interest to maintain the standards of fair and balanced education to the reader. Questions about specific strategies can be directed to the Office of Continuing Medical Education, University of Virginia School of Medicine, Charlottesville, Virginia.

**The authors/editors listed below have identified no professional or financial affiliations for themselves or their spouse/partner:**
Andrea L. Campaigne, MD; Marshall W. Carpenter, MD; Brian M. Casey, MD; Deborah L. Conway, MD (Guest Editor); Donald J. Dudley, MD; J. Seth Hawkins, MD; Moshe Hod, MD; Carla Holloway (Acquisitions Editor); Kelly J. Hunt, PhD; María L. Igarzabal, MD; Siri L. Kjos, MD; Oded Langer MD, PhD; Gustavo Leguizamón, MD; Peter W. Nathanielsz, MD, PhD, ScD, FRCOG; Lucilla Poston PhD, FRCOG; William F. Rayburn, MD (Contributing Editor); E. Albert Reece, MD, PhD, MBA; Alvie C. Richardson, MD; Kelly L. Schuller, PhD; Charanpal Singh, MD; Paul D. Taylor, PhD; and, Yariv Yogev, MD.

**The authors/editors listed below identified the following professional or financial affiliations for themselves or their spouse/partner:**
Lois Jovanovic, MD is an independent contractor, a consultant, and on the advisory committee for Eli Lilly, Novo Nordisk, Dexcom, and Medtronic MiniMed.

*Disclosure of Discussion of non-FDA approved uses for pharmaceutical products and/or medical devices:*
**The University of Virginia School of Medicine, as an ACCME provider, requires that all faculty presenters identify and disclose any "off label" uses for pharmaceutical and medical device products. The University of Virginia School of Medicine recommends that each physician fully review all the available data on new products or procedures prior to instituting them with patients.**

## TO ENROLL

To enroll in the Obstetrics and Gynecology Clinics of North America Continuing Medical Education program, call customer service at 1-800-654-2452 or visit us online at: *www.theclinics.com/home/cme*. The CME program is available to subscribers for an additional fee of $195.00

# CONSULTING EDITOR

**WILLIAM F. RAYBURN, MD,** Seligman Professor and Chair, Department of Obstetrics and Gynecology, University of New Mexico Health Science Center and School of Medicine, Albuquerque, New Mexico

# GUEST EDITOR

**DEBORAH L. CONWAY, MD,** Assistant Professor, Department of Obstetrics and Gynecology, Division of Maternal-Fetal Medicine, and Director–Diabetes in Pregnancy Program, The University of Texas Health Science Center at San Antonio, San Antonio, Texas

# CONTRIBUTORS

**ANDREA L. CAMPAIGNE, MD,** Resident Physician, Department of Obstetrics and Gynecology, The University of Texas Health Science Center at San Antonio, San Antonio, Texas

**MARSHALL W. CARPENTER, MD,** Associate Professor and Director, Division of Maternal Fetal Medicine, Department of Obstetrics and Gynecology, Women and Infants' Hospital of Rhode Island/Brown University School of Medicine, Providence, Rhode Island

**BRIAN M. CASEY, MD,** Associate Professor, Department of Obstetrics and Gynecology, University of Texas Southwestern Medical School, Dallas; Medical Director, Women's Health Centers, Parkland Health and Hospital System, Dallas, Texas

**DEBORAH L. CONWAY, MD,** Assistant Professor, Department of Obstetrics and Gynecology, Division of Maternal-Fetal Medicine, and Director–Diabetes in Pregnancy Program, The University of Texas Health Science Center at San Antonio, San Antonio, Texas

**DONALD J. DUDLEY, MD,** Professor, Department of Obstetrics and Gynecology, University of Texas Health Science Center at San Antonio, San Antonio, Texas

**J. SETH HAWKINS, MD,** Fellow, Maternal–Fetal Medicine, University of Texas Southwestern Medical School

**MOSHE HOD, MD,** Sackler Faculty of Medicine, Perinatal Division, Helen Schneider Hospital for Women, Rabin Medical Center, Tel Aviv University, Israel

**KELLY J. HUNT, PhD,** Assistant Professor, Department of Biostatistics, Bioinformatics and Epidemiology, Medical University of South Carolina, Charleston, South Carolina

MARÍA L. IGARZABAL, MD, Assitant Professor, Postgraduate Program in Medical Genetics, Department of Obstetrics and Gynecology, Center for Medical Education and Clinical Research (C.E.M.I.C.) University, Buenos Aires, Argentina

LOIS JOVANOVIC, MD, Sansum Diabetes Research Institute, Santa Barbara, California

SIRI L. KJOS, MD, Department of Obstetrics and Gynecology, Harbor UCLA Medical Center, Torrance, California

ODED LANGER, MD, PhD, Professor and Chairman, Department of Obstetrics and Gynecology, St. Luke's-Roosevelt Hospital Center, Women's Health Service, University Hospital of Columbia University, New York, New York

GUSTAVO LEGUIZAMÓN, Postgraduate Professor in Obstetrics and Gynecology, Department of Obstetrics and Gynecology, Center for Medical Education and Clinical Research (C.E.M.I.C.) University, Buenos Aires, Argentina

PETER W. NATHANIELSZ, MD, PhD, ScD, FRCOG, Professor and Director, Department of Obstetrics & Gynecology, Center for Pregnancy and Newborn Research, The University of Texas of Health Science Center, San Antonio, Texas

LUCILLA POSTON, PhD, FRCOG, Professor, Maternal and Fetal Unit, Department of Women's Health, Division of Reproduction and Endocrinology, King's College London, St. Thomas' Hospital, London, UK

E. ALBERT REECE, MD, PhD, MBA, Vice President for Medical Affairs, University of Maryland; John Z. and Akiko K. Bowers Distinguished Professor and Dean, School of Medicine, Baltimore, Maryland

ALVIE C. RICHARDSON, MD, Fellow, Division of Maternal Fetal Medicine, Department of Obstetrics and Gynecology, Women and Infants' Hospital of Rhode Island/Brown University School of Medicine, Providence, Rhode Island

KELLY L. SCHULLER, PhD, Department of Biostatistics, Bioinformatics and Epidemiology, Medical University of South Carolina, Charleston, South Carolina

CHARANPAL SINGH, MD, Sansum Diabetes Research Institute, Santa Barbara, California

PAUL D. TAYLOR, PhD, Lecturer, Maternal and Fetal Unit, Department of Women's Health, Division of Reproduction and Endocrinology, King's College London, St. Thomas' Hospital, London, UK

YARIV YOGEV, MD, Sackler Faculty of Medicine, Perinatal Division, Helen Schneider Hospital for Women, Rabin Medical Center, Tel Aviv University, Israel

# CONTENTS

> The authors review studies published in the past 10 years that examine the prevalence and trends in the prevalence of gestational diabetes mellitus (GDM). The prevalence of GDM in a population is reflective of the prevalence of type 2 diabetes within that population. In low-risk populations, such as those found in Sweden, the prevalence in population-based studies is lower than 2% even when universal testing is offered, whereas studies in high-risk populations, such as the Native American Cree, Northern Californian Hispanics, and Northern Californian Asians, reported prevalence rates ranging from 4.9% to 12.8%. Prevalence rates for GDM obtained from hospital-based studies similarly reflect the risk of type 2 diabetes in a population with a single hospital-based study in Australia reporting prevalences ranging from 3.0% in Anglo-Celtic women to 17.0% in Indian women. Finally, of the eight studies published that report on trends in the prevalence of GDM, six report an increase in the prevalence of GDM across most racial/ethnic groups studied. In summary, diabetes during pregnancy is a common and increasing complication of pregnancy.

> The developed and developing worlds are experiencing an epidemic of obesity and associated predisposition to diabetes. This

epidemic places a major drain on health care resources. It is now clear that maternal obesity and gestational diabetes have major adverse effects on the developing fetus that lead to increased neonatal morbidity and mortality, as discussed elsewhere in this issue. Obesity in pregnancy and gestational diabetes represent a special problem, not only as a result of their immediate adverse effects on maternal health and pregnancy outcome, but also because of growing evidence for their persistent and deleterious effects on the developing child.

## FORTHCOMING ISSUES

## RECENT ISSUES

---

**The Clinics are now available online!**
http://www.theclinics.com

---

ELSEVIER
SAUNDERS

Obstet Gynecol Clin N Am
34 (2007) xiii–xiv

OBSTETRICS AND
GYNECOLOGY
CLINICS
OF NORTH AMERICA

# Foreword

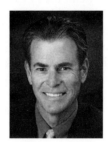

William F. Rayburn, MD
*Consulting Editor*

Diabetes mellitus represents one of the most challenging medical complications during pregnancy. This issue of the *Obstetrics and Gynecology Clinics of North America*, edited by Deborah Conway, MD, provides an overview of current understandings and management guidelines about diabetes during pregnancy. Because few well-designed studies are performed during pregnancy, many of the guidelines described here are based on expert and consensus opinions by this very qualified group of authors.

Approximately 90% of diabetes cases encountered during pregnancy are gestational-onset. Gestational diabetes is one of the most common clinical conditions facing obstetricians and their patients. Its reported prevalence in the United States ranges from 1% to 14%, with 2% to 5% being the most common figure during pregnancy. *Gestational* implies that this carbohydrate intolerance disorder is induced by pregnancy, perhaps from exaggerated physiologic changes in glucose metabolism. An alternative explanation is that gestational diabetes is maturity-onset or type 2 diabetes unmasked or discovered during pregnancy. More than half of women with gestational diabetes ultimately develop overt type 2 diabetes in the ensuing 20 years, and there is mounting evidence for long-range complications that include obesity and diabetes among their offspring.

More than 8 million women in the United States have pregestational diabetes mellitus, and it is observed in 1% of all pregnancies. Pregestational diabetes is classified as to whether insulin is required (type 1) or not required (type 2) to avoid ketoacidosis. The rapidly increasing incidence of type 2 pregestational diabetes mellitus is caused, in part, by an increased prevalence of

0889-8545/07/$ - see front matter © 2007 Published by Elsevier Inc.
doi:10.1016/j.ogc.2007.05.001

*obgyn.theclinics.com*

obesity. Unlike gestational diabetes, overt diabetes has a more clearly significant impact on pregnancy outcome. The embryo, as well as the fetus and mother, can experience serious complications directly from diabetes. The likelihood of successful pregnancy outcomes are related somewhat to the degree of glucose control, but more importantly to the intensity of any underlying maternal cardiovascular or renal disease.

The distinguished authors assembled in this issue bring their expertise to promote diabetes self-management, describe intrapartum considerations for safe delivery, and educate about health care considerations beyond pregnancy. Management of diabetic problems involves the following components: (1) new treatment and monitoring modalities, (2) efficacy and safety of insulin analogues and oral hypoglycemic medications, (3) preventing or detecting excess fetal growth, and (4) reducing adverse events with delivery. These interventions are multifaceted for the highest quality of care to be delivered by the obstetrician-gynecologist.

William F. Rayburn, MD
*Department of Obstetrics and Gynecology*
*University of New Mexico School of Medicine*
*MSC10 5580 1 University of New Mexico*
*Albuquerque, NM 87131-0001, USA*

*E-mail address:* wrayburn@salud.unm.edu

ELSEVIER
SAUNDERS

Obstet Gynecol Clin N Am
34 (2007) xv–xvi

OBSTETRICS AND
GYNECOLOGY
CLINICS
OF NORTH AMERICA

# Preface

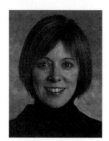

Deborah L. Conway, MD
*Guest Editor*

The basic and clinical science of diabetes mellitus is making rapid strides toward improved understanding, care, and cure. Many of these advances affect our management of the pregnant woman with diabetes, but as busy care providers, we are hard-pressed to keep up with these changes. As conscientious medical practitioners, we often wonder if the latest news from the world of diabetes research can be safely and effectively applied in the setting of pregnancy. How can we augment the core principles we espouse—promotion of diabetes self-management, normalization of blood glucose levels, a safe delivery for the mother and the infant, and patient education about future risks to the woman with diabetes and her offspring—with new information that benefits our patients?

The authors who have contributed to this issue of the *Obstetrics & Gynecology Clinics of North America* have some answers to that question. We start out with a broad view provided by Hunt and Schuller, looking at the increasing prevalence of diabetes in pregnancy. The impact of this increasing prevalence is made more urgent by the review by Nathanielsz, Poston, and Taylor describing the effects on long-term health of being exposed to diabetes and obesity *in utero*. Richardson and Carpenter explain the emerging evidence connecting diabetes with inflammation, mediators of which can have far-reaching adverse health effects. These are emerging topics that will frame how we think about and take care of diabetes in the future, from basic science to public health policy.

Moving into clinical care, the importance of excellent periconceptional diabetes management is described by Leguizamón, Igarzabal, and Reece.

0889-8545/07/$ - see front matter © 2007 Published by Elsevier Inc.
doi:10.1016/j.ogc.2007.04.005     *obgyn.theclinics.com*

The use of new treatment and monitoring modalities are discussed by Drs. Yogev and Hod, and the safety and efficacy of oral anti-diabetic agents and insulin analogs in pregnancy are discussed by Langer and Singh and Jovanovic, respectively. The most-feared complication of diabetes in pregnancy, the occurrence of stillbirth, is explored by Dudley. Strategies for the prevention and detection of the most frequent complication of diabetes in pregnancy, excessive fetal growth, are reviewed by Campaigne and Conway, and Hawkins and Casey provide an evidence-based approach to managing labor and delivery in women with diabetes. Finally, because women spend much more of their lives not pregnant, we conclude with an essential review by Kjos of the postnatal care of these women, focusing on the high lifetime risk of type 2 diabetes in women with gestational diabetes, and how to modify this risk. Keeping this in focus benefits not only these women, but their current and future offspring as well.

I am profoundly grateful to the dedicated and gifted individuals who have contributed to this issue. Each article was provided by true leaders in their respective topics, and I very much appreciate their willingness, even eagerness, to participate—though it came as no surprise to me, because their dedication to the highest quality care of pregnant women with diabetes has been inspiring my efforts for many, many years.

Deborah L. Conway, MD
*Division of Maternal Fetal Medicine*
*Department of Obstetrics and Gynecology*
*University of Texas Health Science Center—San Antonio*
*7703 Floyd Curl Drive*
*San Antonio, TX 78229, USA*

*E-mail address:* conway@uthscsa.edu

ELSEVIER
SAUNDERS

Obstet Gynecol Clin N Am
34 (2007) 173–199

OBSTETRICS AND
GYNECOLOGY
CLINICS
OF NORTH AMERICA

# The Increasing Prevalence of Diabetes in Pregnancy

Kelly J. Hunt, PhD*, Kelly L. Schuller, PhD

*Department of Biostatistics, Bioinformatics and Epidemiology,
Medical University of South Carolina, 135 Cannon Street,
Suite 303, Charleston, SC 29425, USA*

As the incidence of diabetes continues to rise and increasingly affects individuals of all ages including young adults and children, women of childbearing age are at increased risk of diabetes during pregnancy [1–7]. The lifetime risk of diabetes among the cohort of individuals born in the United States in 2000 was estimated to be 33% in males and 39% in females, based on information obtained from the National Health and Nutrition Examination Surveys (NHANES) conducted 1984 to 2000 [8]. Moreover, the estimated lifetime risk of diabetes was higher at birth and throughout life for ethnic and racial minority groups than for non-Hispanic whites and for women when compared with men [8]. The estimated lifetime diabetes risk at birth ranged from 31.2% in non-Hispanic white women to 52.5% in Hispanic women, and from 26.7% in non-Hispanic white men to 45.4% in Hispanic men [8].

The epidemic of diabetes is not limited to western countries, but reaches worldwide affecting individuals in countries such as India and China [9–11]. A recent study estimates the global prevalence of diabetes in 2000 at 2.8%, translating into 171 million individuals who have diabetes, and projects that in 2030 the prevalence will be 4.4%, translating into 366 million individuals who have diabetes worldwide [9]. The increased prevalence is attributed to the aging population structure, urbanization, the obesity epidemic, and physical inactivity.

At first glance, the obesity epidemic driven by changes in lifestyle seems to be the driving force behind the increased prevalence of diabetes. The current

* Corresponding author.
*E-mail address:* huntke@musc.edu (K.J. Hunt).

0889-8545/07/$ - see front matter © 2007 Elsevier Inc. All rights reserved.
doi:10.1016/j.ogc.2007.03.002                                    *obgyn.theclinics.com*

epidemic of obesity and overweight is widespread, affecting both children and adults of many ethnic backgrounds in North America and internationally [12,13]. In each consecutive NHANES survey starting with NHANES I, conducted from 1971 to 1974, through completion of the most recent NHANES survey cycle, conducted from 1999 to 2002, there has been a marked increase in the prevalence of obesity in children and adults across all ethnic, gender, and age strata [14–18]. In contrast to diabetes, where both men and women of minority populations are affected disproportionately, minority women but not men tend to be disproportionately obese. The prevalence of obesity ranged from 50% in non-Hispanic black women to 30% in non-Hispanic white women in NHANES conducted 1999 to 2000 [16]. In contrast, in men the prevalence was 27% in non-Hispanic white men, 29% in Mexican American men, and 28% in non-Hispanic black men [16].

Traditionally, epidemiologic studies of risk factors associated with type 2 diabetes had focused on adults and characteristics of adult study participants. However, early life exposures are emerging as potentially important risk factors. The "fetal origin of disease" hypothesis proposes that gestational programming may critically influence adult health and disease [19]. Gestational programming is a process whereby stimuli or stresses that occur at critical or sensitive periods of development permanently change structure, physiology, and metabolism, which predispose individuals to disease in adult life [20]. Many animal studies provide support for gestational programming, as do epidemiologic studies of the Dutch Hunger Winter and the "thrifty phenotype" hypothesis, which proposes that low birth weight, indicative of poor prenatal nutrition, has an effect on development that manifests itself later in life as an increased risk for several chronic diseases [21–36].

In contrast to times of famine, today the intrauterine environment is more likely to expose the fetus to hyperglycemia or excess energy. Obesity before pregnancy, and high weight gain during pregnancy, predispose women to gestational diabetes mellitus (GDM) and early onset type 2 diabetes [37–40]. Maternal diabetes during gestation exposes the fetus to hyperglycemia, resulting in increased fetal insulin levels that promote the storage of excess energy as fat and act as a growth factor. Exposure to maternal diabetes early in pregnancy is associated with birth defects, and later in pregnancy is associated with high birth weight, increased childhood and adult obesity, and increased risk of type 2 diabetes [41–48]. Children exposed *in utero* to maternal diabetes are at higher risk of obesity and diabetes than their unexposed siblings, suggesting that the increased risk to the exposed offspring is not exclusively genetic [49,50]. In the Pima Indians, the population with the highest known rate of diabetes, a study found that the increased exposure to diabetes *in utero* and increased weight in children accounted for most of the increased prevalence of diabetes over the past 30 years in Pima Indian children [42].

If the diabetic intrauterine environment is substantially contributing to the obesity and diabetes epidemics, not only will the prevalence continue to increase across all populations, but populations that have a high prevalence of diabetes, such as non-Hispanic blacks and Mexican Americans, will continue to be disproportionately affected by these epidemics, resulting in a perpetual widening of health disparities between racial and ethnic groups. For these reasons, it is imperative to understand the transgenerational epidemiology and etiology of diabetes and develop simple, economical, and effective prevention strategies. Because the prevalence of diagnosed diabetes (either type 1 or type 2) before pregnancy is addressed in studies of the increasing prevalence of diabetes, the current review is focused on GDM defined as glucose intolerance with onset or first recognition during pregnancy. GDM is a common complication of pregnancy and often a precursor of type 2 diabetes. Therefore, the authors' objectives were to review studies examining the prevalence of GDM as well as studies examining trends in the prevalence of GDM. In this context, the authors also review the diagnostic criteria for diabetes and GDM and their changes over time.

## Methods

### Literature search

A literature search was conducted in MEDLINE using the following search criteria: "gestational diabetes" as a MeSH term or text word, combined with "epidemiology" as a subheading or MeSH term, "prevalence" as a MeSH term, or "trend" or "screening" as a text word. In addition, the search was limited to English-language articles published in the last 10 years (July 1st, 1996 through October 1st, 2006). These search criteria yielded 1025 articles. The lead author (KJH) reviewed either the abstract or title of these articles to determine if they were suitable to assess either the current prevalence of GDM or trends in the prevalence of GDM. The review was limited to population-based studies that included at least 500 pregnant women, or hospital-based studies that included at least 1000 pregnant women with at least 70% of the population being screened for GDM. In addition, articles that assessed GDM trends were required to span at least 3 years. When multiple articles were published on a single population, the article containing the most recent information was retained. In addition to conducting the literature search, reference lists of review articles obtained from the MEDLINE search were reviewed for additional pertinent studies.

### Diabetes and gestational diabetes mellitus, screening, and definitions

The definition of diabetes has changed over the past 10 years. Box 1 [51] summarizes the definitions of diabetes commonly employed in recent epidemiologic literature.

Although the 1985 and 1999 World Health Organization (WHO) criteria require a 2-hour 75-g oral glucose tolerance test (OGTT), the 1997

---

**Box 1. Definitions of diabetes commonly employed in recent epidemiologic literature**

*World Health Organization (WHO), 1985* [51]
Fasting glucose greater than or equal to 140 or a 2-hour 75-g oral glucose tolerance test (OGTT) glucose greater than or equal to 200

*WHO, 1999* [116]
Fasting glucose greater than or equal 126 or a 2-hour 75-g OGTT glucose greater than or equal to 200

*American Diabetes Association (ADA), 1997* [115]
Focused on a fasting glucose greater than or equal to 126, but also recognizes a casual or 2-hr 75-g OGGT greater than or equal to 200; therefore, epidemiologic studies based on the ADA criteria may be based exclusively on fasting glucose levels or include information from a 2-hr 75-g OGTT.

---

All criteria are stated in mg/dL and use venous plasma.

---

American Diabetes Association (ADA) criteria are focused on fasting glucose, but also recognize a casual or 2-hour 75-g OGTT glucose level greater than or equal to 200 mg/dL as diagnostic of diabetes. Therefore, epidemiologic studies based on the ADA criteria may be based exclusively on fasting glucose levels or include information from an OGTT.

The recommended definition of GDM and criteria identifying who should be screened for GDM has varied widely across populations and over time; therefore, the authors review screening criteria and diagnostic criteria for GDM employed in recent epidemiologic literature. Table 1 [52–54] summarizes screening criteria, whereas Table 2 [55,56] summarizes widely accepted GDM diagnostic criteria. In summary, recommended screening ranges from selective screening of average- and high-risk individuals to universal diagnostic testing of the entire population dependent on the risk of diabetes in the population.

The diagnostic criteria for GDM have evolved over time and are not agreed upon internationally; therefore, definitions of GDM used in the epidemiologic literature vary considerably. Notably, at the 4th International Workshop Conference on GDM, it was agreed that the Carpenter and Coustan [57] (C&C) criteria should replace the National Diabetes Data Group [58] (NDDG) criteria, resulting in a significant lowering of the thresholds and an increase in the prevalence of GDM. Because several organizations currently endorse the C&C criteria [59–61], for consistency throughout the review, the authors refer to the C&C criteria or to the NDDG criteria when they are used in different references.

Table 1
Gestational diabetes mellitus screening criteria

|  | Target population | Recommended screening test |
| --- | --- | --- |
| WHO, 1985 and 1999 Reports of the WHO Consultation on the Diagnosis and Classification of Diabetes Mellitus [51,116] | Not specified | Nonhigh risk: diagnostic 2 h 75 g OGTT at 24–28 wk of gestation High risk: also test early in pregnancy |
| EASD, 1991 [52] | Universal | A random blood glucose ≥ 108 when fasting or 2 h after food or ≥ 126 when within 2 h of food at initial prenatal visit and 28 wk gestation |
| ACOG, 1994 [53] | From universal to selective, dependent upon the risk of diabetes in the population | Nonhigh risk: 1 h 50 g GCT ≥ 140 or ≥ 130 OR diagnostic 3 h 100 g OGTT at 24–28 wk of gestation High risk: also screen as early as possible in pregnancy |
| ADA, 1997 [115] | "Low-risk[a]" women do not need to be screened | 1 h 50 g GCT ≥ 140 at 24–28 wk of gestation |
| ADA [59] and ACOG [60], post 1997 4th International Workshop Conference on GDM [61] | Selective: "Low-risk[b]" women do not need to be screened | Average risk: 1 h 50 g GCT ≥140 or ≥130 at 24–28 wk of gestation OR diagnostic 2 h 75 g OGTT High risk: also screen as early as possible in pregnancy |
| ADIPS, 1998 [54] | Universal | 1 h 50 g GCT ≥ 140 OR 1 h 75 g GCT ≥ 144 at 26–28 wk of gestation |

All criteria use venous plasma.

*Abbreviations:* ACOG, American College of Obstetricians and Gynecologists; ADIPS, Australasian Diabetes in Pregnancy Society; EASD, European Association for the Study of Diabetes; GCT, glucose challenge test.

[a] The ADA (1997) initially defined "low risk" as women meeting the four following criteria: (1) age less than 25, (2) not a member of an ethnic group with a high prevalence for diabetes (eg, not Hispanic, Native American/Alaskan, Asian/Pacific Islander, African American), (3) normal prepregnancy body weight (not 20% or more over desired body weight or BMI 27 kg/m2 or more), and (4) no family history of diabetes in first-degree relatives.

[b] At the 1997 4th International Workshop Conference on GDM, the following two criteria were added to the "low risk" definition: (5) no history of poor obstetric outcome, and (6) no history of abnormal glucose tolerance.

## Results

### Population-based studies

For purposes of this review, population-based studies were defined as studies that attempted to include a representative sample of the general population in a defined geographic area. Moreover, because the focus for

Table 2
Gestational diabetes mellitus diagnostic criteria

| | Load (g) | Duration (hours) | Abnormal values (n) | Fasting, 1-, 2- and 3-hour OGTT thresholds (mg/dL) |
|---|---|---|---|---|
| O'Sullivan and Mahan[a], 1964 [55] | 100 | 3 | ≥2 | 90, 165, 145, 125 |
| NDDG, 1979 [58] ACOG, 1994 [53] ADA, 1997 [115] | 100 | 3 | ≥2 | 105, 190, 165, 145 |
| C&C, 1982 [57] | 100 | 3 | ≥2 | 95, 180, 155, 140 |
| JSOG, 1984 [56] | 75 | 2 | ≥2 | 100, 180, 150 |
| WHO, 1985 [51] | 75 | 2 | ≥1 | 140, N/A, 140 |
| EASD, 1991 [52] | 75 | 2 | ≥1 | 108, N/A, 162 |
| ADA [59] and ACOG [60], post 1997 4th International | 75 or | 2 | ≥2 | 95, 180, 155 |
| Workshop Conference on GDM [61] | 100 | 3 | ≥2 | 95, 180, 155, 140 |
| WHO, 1999 [116] | 75 | 2 | ≥1 | N/A, N/A, 140 |
| ADIPS, 1998 [54] | 75 | 2 | ≥1 | 99, N/A, 144 |

*Abbreviations:* ADIPS, Australasian Diabetes in Pregnancy Society; C&C, Carpenter and Coustan; EASD, European Association for the Study of Diabetes; JSOG, Japanese Society of Obstetrics and Gynecology; NDDG, National Diabetes Data Group.

[a] All criteria use venous plasma except for O'Sullivan and Mahan, which was defined using whole venous blood.

population-based studies was having a representative study population, universal screening or testing for GDM was not required for inclusion in the review. Population-based studies of more than 500 individuals are summarized in Table 3. The prevalence of GDM varied depending upon the diagnostic criteria employed in the study; whether the study was retrospective or prospective; the source of the study data; as well as the country of residence, ethnicity, and racial group of the study participants. In general, the authors observed lower prevalence rates in retrospective studies using pre-existing databases or routinely collected health statistics where a clear screening policy for GDM was not in place [62–67], compared with retrospective or prospective studies that report universal screening for GDM.

In studies conducted in North America, the observed prevalence was higher in Asians, African Americans, Native North Americans from Canada, and Hispanics than in non-Hispanic whites [38,63,64,68–72]. In a retrospective cohort study of the Kaiser Permanente Medical Care Group of Northern California, where 93.5% of the population was screened for GDM, the prevalence ranged from 2.5% in white women to 5.7% in Asian women using the NDDG criteria, and from 3.9% in white women to 8.3% in Asian women using the C&C criteria [68]. In the Nurses Health Study II, which relied on self-reported diagnosis, the observed prevalence was over 10% in African Americans (10.6%) and Asians (10.5%), and approximately 5% in whites (4.8%) [38]. Finally, in retrospective studies conducted in

Native North Americans in Canada, the prevalence based on NDDG crite-ria ranged from 8.4% to 12.8% [64,70–72]. The single study conducted in South America was a prospective study conducted in Brazil in a diverse pop-ulation and reported a prevalence of 2.4% based on ADA [59] criteria using the 2-hour 75-g OGTT diagnostic criteria, and 7.2% based on WHO criteria [73].

Population-based studies conducted in northern Europe used a 2-hour 75-g OGGT to diagnose GDM; however, varying diagnostic cutpoints were employed. Using the 2-hour 75-g OGTT, observed prevalence rates in the United Kingdom, Holland, Sweden, and Denmark ranged from 0.6% in Dutch women to 3.6% using local criteria in a Danish population [65,66,74–78]. In two studies conducted in Italy, a 3-hour 100-g OGTT using the C&C criteria following universal screening was employed to diagnose GDM. In the earlier study conducted in northwest Tuscany, the prevalence was 6.3% [79], whereas in the later study conducted in a volunteer popula-tion in Sardinia, the prevalence was 22.3% [80].

Reported prevalence rates in population-based studies in Turkey, Iran, Bahrain, Ethiopia, and India ranged from 1.2% in Turkey (NDDG criteria following universal screening) to 15.5% in Bahraini women (C&C with a 3-hour 75-g OGTT following universal screening) [81–86]. In a retrospective study in Australia, which included all singleton deliveries in Victoria in 1996 and used routinely collected information in two databases, the prevalence was 3.6% in non-Aboriginal women and 4.3% in Aboriginal women [67]. In a study conducted in six urban districts in Tianjin, China, using 1999 WHO diagnostic criteria and universal screening, the prevalence was 2.3% [87]. Finally, in a study conducted in Japan, using the Japanese Society of Obstetrics and Gynecology (JSOG) criteria for GDM and universal screening, the prevalence was 2.9% [88].

*Hospital-based studies*

Hospital-based studies of more than 1000 unselected individuals, where universal screening or testing was employed and at least 70% of the popu-lation was screened for GDM, are summarized in Table 4. Similar to the population-based studies, in the hospital-based studies, the prevalence of GDM varied depending upon the diagnostic criteria employed in the study, whether the study was retrospective or prospective as well as the country of residence, ethnicity, and racial group of the study participants. Three of the hospital-based studies directly compare GDM prevalence rates based on NDDG and C&C criteria [89–91]. In these three studies, NDDG rates range from 3.2% in a study conducted in Mexico [89] to 8.8% in a study con-ducted in Spain [90], with corresponding C&C rates ranging from 4.1% to 11.6% [89–91].

The hospital-based studies conducted in the United States diagnosed GDM based on a 3-hour OGTT and report prevalence rates ranging from

Table 3
Prevalence of GDM in population-based studies

| Author | Screening criteria | GDM criteria | Time frame | Source population | Country | Ethnic group; n | Prevalence |
|---|---|---|---|---|---|---|---|
| Rosenberg, 2005 [62] | Varied depending upon prenatal care received | | Retrospective; 1991–2001 | Live singleton New York City births with birth certificate data on prepregnancy weight and weight gain | USA | NHB, 86,908; NHW, 96,581; NHA, 38,570; Hispanic, 107,612 | 3.7%, total; 3.7%, NHB; 2.6%, NHW; 6.6%, NHA; 3.5%, Hispanic |
| Ferrara, 2002 [68] | Universal screening at 24–28 wk; 1 h 50 g GCT ≥ 140; 93.5% screened | C&C; NDDG | Retrospective; 1996 | Kaiser Permanente Medical Care Group of Northern California; computerized hospitalization records | USA | White, 13,714; AA, 2345; Hispanic, 5026; Asian; 4121 | NDDG and C&C: 3.2 and 4.8%, total; 2.5 and 3.9%, White; 2.6 and 3.4%, AA; 3.4 and 4.9%, Hispanic; 5.7 and 8.3%, Asian |
| Kieffer, 2001 [69] | Universal screening at 24–28 wk; 1 h 50 g GCT ≥ 140; 98.9% of Latinas and 96.6% of AA screened | NDDG | Retrospective; 1995–1998 | Latina and AA women who received at least 4 prenatal care visits in large Detroit health system; medical record surveys | USA | Latina, 653; AA, 552 | 5.4%, Latina; 3.9%, AA |
| Williams, 1999 [63] | Varied depending upon prenatal care received | | Retrospective; 1987–1995 | Mothers born in Washington State since 1949 delivering a singleton birth between 1987–1995; vital records and hospital discharge summaries | USA | NHW, 21,528; AA, 6359; Native American, 7456; Hispanic, 6496 | 2.8%, NHW; 2.6%, AA; 2.7%, Native American; 3.0%, Hispanic |
| Solomon, 1997 [38] | Varied depending upon prenatal care received; self-reported diagnosis | | Prospective; 1989–1994 | Nurses' Health Study II women with singleton pregnancies and no history of diabetes or GDM | USA | White, 13,771; AA, 113; Hispanic, 224; Asian, 248 | 4.9%, total: 4.8%; White; 10.6%, AA; 7.6%, Hispanic; 10.5%, Asian |

| Reference | Screening | Criteria | Study design; years | Setting | Country | Population | Prevalence |
|---|---|---|---|---|---|---|---|
| Rodrigues, 1999 [70,71] | Universal screening at 24–30 wk; 1 h 50 g GCT ≥ 140 | NDDG | Retrospective; 1995–1996 | Cree: 9 communities in James Bay, Quebec; maternal medical charts Non-Native: Royal Victoria Hospital, Montreal; McGill Obstetric and Neonatal Database | Canada | Cree, 579; Non-Native, 7718 | 12.8%, Cree; 5.3%, Non-Native |
| Godwin, 1999 [64] | Varied depending upon prenatal care received; GDM was defined according to NDDG criteria or a fasting or 1 h 50 g GCT ≥ 140 with physician diagnosis | | Retrospective; 1987–1995 | Weeneebayko Hosptial, Moose Factory, James Bay, Ontario; chart review | Canada | Native Swampy Cree, 1298 | 8.5% |
| Harris, 1997 [72] | Universal screening at 24–28 wk; 1 h 50 g GCT ≥ 140; 90% screened | NDDG | Retrospective; 1990–1993 | Sioux Lookout Zone, Northwestern Ontario; medical records | Canada | Native Ojibwa-Cree, 741 | 8.4% |
| Schmidt, 2001 [73] | Universal Testing at 24–28 wk; 2 h 75 g OGTT; ADA, post 1997 and WHO, 1999 including 0 h≥ 126 | | Prospective; 1991–1995 | General prenatal care clinics in the National Health Service | Brazil | White, 2234; AA, 679; Mixed, 2042; Other, 21 | 2.4%, ADA 7.2%, WHO |
| Janghorbani, 2006 [65] | Universal screening at 26–28 wk or high-risk testing; random plasma glucose ≥ 117 | 2hr 75 g OGTT; 0 h ≥ 108; 2 h ≥ 140 | Retrospective; 1996–1997 | Plymouth, southwest UK; databases and midwifery care notes | UK | NHW; 4942 | 1.8% |
| Weijers, 1998 [66] | Varied depending upon prenatal care received; medical history of physician-diagnosed GDM | | Retrospective; 1992–1997 | Town borough of Amsterdam; physician-diagnosed GDM reported in hospital registration | Holland | Dutch, 483; Non-Dutch, 1157 | 0.6%, Dutch; 2.6%, Non-Dutch |

(continued on next page)

Table 3 (continued)

| Author | Screening criteria | GDM criteria | Time frame | Source population | Country | Ethnic group; n | Prevalence |
|---|---|---|---|---|---|---|---|
| Ostlund, 2003, 2004 [74,75] | Universal testing offered at 28–32 wk; 73.5% accepted: EASD (0 h ≥ 121 cut-point) | | Prospective; 1994–1996 | Defined geographical area of Sweden | Sweden | Nordic, 3211; Non-Nordic, 405 | 1.7% |
| Aberg, 2002 [76] | Universal testing offered at 27–28 wk with additional testing in high-risk patients; not clear what percentage of the population accepted; 2 h 75 g OGTT ≥ 162 whole-blood | | Prospective; 1995–1997 | Lund University Hospital | Sweden | Not specified; 12,382 | 1.2% |
| Jensen, 2003 [77] | Universal testing offered, high risk—early in pregnancy and at 28–32 wk; EASD (0 h ≥ 111 and 2 h ≥ 164 whole-blood) | | Prospective; 1999–2000 | 4 Danish health care centers | Denmark | Not specified; (5235 using 56.2% imputed values) | 2.4% |
| Kvetny, 1999 [78] | High risk[b] testing at 24–28 weeks; 2 h 75 g OGTT ≥ 121 or WHO, 1999; 19.5% tested | | Prospective; 1995–1997 | Ribe county prenatal care patients | Denmark | Not specified; 6158 | 3.6%, local criteria; 2.8%, WHO |
| Murgia, 2006 [80] | Universal screening at 16–18, 24–26, and 30–32 wk; 1 h 50 g GCT ≥ 130 | C&C | Prospective; 2006[a] | Sardinian volunteers | Italy | Sardinian; 1103 | 22.3% |
| Di Cianni, 1997 [79] | Universal screening at 24–28 wk or earlier when high risk; 1 h 50 g GCT ≥ 140 | C&C | Prospective; 1997[a] | 8 health care districts in north-west Tuscany | Italy | Not specified, 2000 | 6.3% |
| Erem, 2003 [81] | Universal screening at 24–28 wk; 1 h 50 g GCT ≥ 140 | NDDG | Prospective; 2003[a] | Central Province of Trabzon City: 7 health stations | Turkey | Not specified, 807 | 1.2% |

| Keshavarz, 2005 [82] | Universal screening high risk— initial visit and at 24–28 wk; 1 h 50 g GCT ≥ 130 | ADA, post 1997 | Prospective; 1999–2001 | Fatemiyeh Hospital in Shahrood City | Iran | Not specified, 1310 | 4.8% |
|---|---|---|---|---|---|---|---|
| Hadaegh, 2005 [83] | Universal screening at 24–28 wk; 1 h 50 g GCT ≥ 130 | C&C and NDDG | Prospective; 2002–2004 | All pregnant women referred to the obstetrics clinics in various parts of Bandar Abbas city | Iran | Not specified (800 using 12.5% imputed values) | 8.1%, NDDG; 11.4%, C&C |
| Al Mahroos, 2005 [84] | Universal screening at 24–28 wk; 1 h 50 g GCT ≥ 140 | C&C with a 3 h 75 g OGTT | Prospective, 2001–2002 | Antenatal clinics at health centers and at Salmaniya Medical Complex | Bahrain | Bahraini, 7575; Expatriate, 2920 | 13.3%, total; 15.5%, Bahraini; 7.5%, Expatriate |
| Seyoum, 1999 [85] | Universal testing after 24 wk; WHO, 1999 | | Prospective; 1999[a] | Women over 24 weeks gestational age; community-based, eastern zone of Tigray | Ethiopia | Not specified; 890 | 3.7% |
| Zargar, 2004 [86] | Universal screening 2nd or 3rd trimester; 1 h 50 g GCT ≥ 140 | Group A: C&C; Group B: WHO, 1999 | Prospective; 1999–2002 | 6 districts of Kashmir valley | India | Not specified; Group A, 1000; Group B, 1000 | 3.1%, Group A; 4.4%, Group B |
| Stone, 2002 [67] | Varied depending upon prenatal care received | | Retrospective; 1996 | Singleton pregnancies for Victoria in 1996; Routinely collected data in Victoria from Perinatal Morbidity Statistics System and Victorian Inpatient Minimum Dataset Data | Australia | Aboriginal, 438; Non-Aboriginal, 59,962 | 3.6%, total; 4.3%, Aboriginal; 3.6%, Non-Aboriginal |

(continued on next page)

Table 3 (*continued*)

| Author | Screening criteria | GDM criteria | Time frame | Source population | Country | Ethnic group: n | Prevalence |
|---|---|---|---|---|---|---|---|
| Yang, 2002 [87] | Universal screening at 26–30 wk; 1 h 50 g GCT ≥ 140 | WHO, 1999 including 0 h ≥ 126 | Prospective; 1998–1999 | 6 urban districts in Tianjin | China | Not specified; 9471 | 2.3% |
| Maegawa, 2003 [88] | Universal screening during first trimester; 1 h 50 g GCT ≥ 130 | JSOG | Prospective; 1999–2001 | 11 hospitals in Mie prefecture or Hiroshima Municipal Asa Hospital | Japan | Japanese; 749 | 2.9% |

*Abbreviations*: AA, African American; EASD, European Association for the Study of Diabetes; GCT, glucose challenge test; JSOG, Japanese Society of Obstetrics and Gynecology; NDDG, National Diabetes Data Group; NHB, non-Hispanic black; NHA, non-Hispanic Asian; NHW, non-Hispanic white.
[a] Indicates that calendar time for participant enrollment was not provided; therefore, the publication date is substituted for the study time frame.
[b] Women who have previous GDM, history of fetal macrosomia, glucosuria, BMI > 29, family history, prior stillbirth, age > 35 y).

2.7% using the NDDG criteria to 6.8% in a largely Mexican American population using the C&C criteria [92–94]. In a Canadian study at the Saskatoon Royal University Hospital, using the NDDG criteria, the prevalence was 11.5% in the Aboriginal population and 3.5% in the non-Aboriginal population [95]. In a study conducted at the University Hospital in Monterrey, Mexico, which compared several diagnostic criteria, the prevalence was 3.2%, 4.1%, and 8.7% based on NDDG, C&C, and 1999 WHO diagnostic criteria, respectively [89]. In Europe, hospital-based studies were conducted in Spain and Italy. Three studies in Spain reported prevalence rates ranging from 3.3% to 8.8% using NDDG criteria [90,96,97]. The two Italian studies report prevalence rates of 4.6% and 8.7% based on C&C criteria [91,98].

Reported prevalence rates in hospital-based studies in Turkey, Iran, Pakistan, India, and Sri Lanka are between 4.1% and 4.7%, with the exception of the study conducted in India, which used the 1999 WHO diagnostic criteria and reports a prevalence of 18.9%, as well as the study conducted in Turkey, which reports a prevalence of 6.6% using the C&C criteria [99–103]. Both hospital-based studies conducted in Australia employed the Australasian Diabetes in Pregnancy Society (ADIPS) criteria, with one reporting an overall prevalence of 5.2% [104] and the second reporting prevalence rates as low as 3.0% in Anglo-Celtic participants and as high as 10.0, 15.0, and 17.0% in Aboriginal, Chinese, and Indian participants, respectively [105]. A single hospital-based study conducted in Japan reported a prevalence of 1.8% based on the JSOG diagnostic criteria [106].

*Trends in the prevalence of gestational diabetes mellitus*

Eight retrospective studies conducted in the past 10 years in the United States, Canada, and Australia examine trends in the prevalence of GDM (Table 5) [107–114]. Three of the four studies conducted in the United States report either universal screening criteria in place and/or evidence of consistent screening in the population, with a screening rate of 96% to 98% in the Kaiser Permanente of Colorado study and 86.8% in the Northern California Kaiser Permanente study [107–109]. Each of the four studies conducted in the United States reports a statistically significant increase in the prevalence of GDM or diabetes during pregnancy in the study period [107–110]. The Kaiser Permanente study conducted in a population representative of the Denver metropolitan area reports a prevalence increase from 2.1% in 1994 to 4.1% in 2002, based on the NDDG diagnostic criteria throughout the study [107]. In addition, they report a greater increase for minorities than whites [107]. Similarly, the Kaiser Permanente study conducted in a population representative of Northern California reports a prevalence increase from 5.1% in 1991 to 7.4% in 1997, which leveled off through 2000 at 6.9% based on the C&C diagnostic criteria [108]. A study conducted on all women who had singleton deliveries in New York city, where universal screening criteria have been practiced since the 1980s, reports a prevalence

Table 4
Prevalence of GDM in hospital-based studies

| Author | Screening criteria | GDM criteria | Time frame | Population/data source[b] | Country | Ethnic group; n | Prevalence |
|---|---|---|---|---|---|---|---|
| Yogev, 2004 [92] | Universal screening at 24-28 wk; 1h 50 g GCT ≥ 130 | C&C | Prospective; 1995–1999 | St. Luke's Roosevelt Hospital Center and University of Texas Health Sciences Center at San Antonio | USA | Mexican American (85%), African American, Caucasian, other; 6857 | 6.8% |
| Stamilio, 2004 [93] | Universal screening at 24-28 wk; 1 h 50 g GCT ≥ 135 | NDDG With 0 h ≥ 100 | Retrospective; 1995–1997 | University of Pennsylvania Medical Center Triple marker screen perinatal database | USA | Not specified; 1825 | 2.7% |
| Danilenko-Dixon, 1999 [94] | Universal screening at 24-30 wk; 1 h 50 g GCT ≥ 140 | NDDG | Retrospective; 1986–1997 | Mayo Clinic, Rochester, MN; perinatal database | USA | White, African American, Asian, Hispanic, other; 18,504 | 3.0% |
| Dyck, 2002 [95] | Universal screening; 1 h 50 g GCT ≥ 140 | NDDG | Prospective; 1998 | Saskatoon Royal University Hospital | Canada | Aboriginal, 252; Non-Aboriginal, 1360 | 11.5%, Aboriginal; 3.5%, Non-Aboriginal |
| Santos-Ayarzagoitia, 2006 [89] | Universal screening; 1 h 50 g GCT ≥ 140 (initial visit); WHO Diagnostic (second visit) | NDDG; C&C; WHO, 1999 | Prospective; 2002–2003 | University Hospital Monterrey, Mexico | Mexico | Does not specify; 1092 | 3.2% NDDG; 4.1%, C&C; 8.7%, WHO |
| Ricart, 2005 [90] | Universal screening at 24-28 wk; 1 h 50 g GCT ≥ 140 | NDDG; C&C | Prospective; 2002 | 16 general hospitals of the Spanish National Health Service | Spain | Caucasian, African, Asian, Caribbean, and other; 9270 | 8.8%, NDDG; 11.6%, C&C |
| Jimenez-Moleon, 2002 [96] | Universal screening; 1 h 50 g GCT ≥ 140 | NDDG | Retrospective; 1995 | Hospital Clinico San Cecilio; abstracted from medical records | Spain | Not specified; 1962 | 3.3% |

| Study | Screening protocol | Criteria | Study type; year | Setting | Country | Ethnicity; N | Prevalence |
|---|---|---|---|---|---|---|---|
| Bartha, 2000 [97] | Universal screening at initial visit and 24–28 wk; 1 h 50 g GCT ≥ 140 | NDDG | Prospective; 2000[a] | University Hospital of Puerto Real | Spain | Not specified; 3986 | 5.9% |
| Di Cianni, 2003 [98] | Universal screening high risk— initial visit and at 24–28 wk; 1 h 50 g GCT ≥ 140 | C&C | Retrospective; 1995–2001 | University of Pisa; data source not given, likely to be medical records | Italy | Italian; 3950 | 8.7% |
| Corrado, 1999 [91] | Universal screening; 1 h 50 g GCT≥135 | NDDG; C&C | Prospective; 1989–1995 | University of Messina and 5 private practices | Italy | Italian; 1000 | 3.4%, NDDG; 4.6%, C&C |
| Yalcin, 1996 [99] | Universal screening at 24–32 wk; 1 h 50 g GCT ≥ 140 | C&C | Prospective; 1996 | Tahir Burak Women's Hospital | Turkey | Turkish; 1000 | 6.6% |
| Larijani, 2003 [100] | Universal screening high risk— initial visit and at 24–28 wk; 1 h 50 g GCT ≥ 130 | C&C | Prospective; 2003[a] | 4 university teaching hospitals in Tehran | Iran | Not specified; 2416 | 4.7% |
| Hassan, 2005 [101] | Universal screening at 24–36 wk; 1 h 50 g GCT ≥ 130 | NDDG | Prospective; 1997 | Lady Reading Hospital | Pakistan | Not specified; 1000 | 4.3% |
| Seshiah, 2004 [102] | Universal screening 2nd or 3rd trimester; 1 h 50 g GCT ≥ 130 | WHO, 1999 including 0 h ≥ 126 | Prospective; 2001 | Raja Sir Ramaswamy Mudhaliar Hospital | India | Not specified; 1251 | 18.9% |
| Wagaarachchi, 2001 [103] | No screening; Universal testing at 24–28 wk | WHO, 1985 | Prospective; 2001[a] | Castle Street Hospital for Women | Sri Lanka | Not specified; 1004 | 4.1% |

(continued on next page)

Table 4 (continued)

| Author | Screening criteria | GDM criteria | Time frame | Population/data source[b] | Country | Ethnic group; n | Prevalence |
|---|---|---|---|---|---|---|---|
| Davey, 2001 [104] | Universal screening at 26–28 wk; 1 h 50 g GCT ≥ 140 | ADIPS | Retrospective; 1996–1998 | Sunshine Hospital, Melbourne; abstracted from medical records | Australia | Not specified; 6032 | 5.2% |
| Yue, 1996 [105] | Universal screening at 24–28 wk; 1 h 50 g GCT ≥ 140 | ADIPS | Prospective; 1996[a] | Royal Prince Alfred Hospital | Australia | Anglo-Celtic, Chinese, Vietnamese, Indian, Arab, Aboriginal; 5243 | 3.0%, Anglo-Celtic; 15.0%, Chinese; 9.0%, Vietnamese; 17.0%, Indian; 7.0%, Arab; 10.0%, Aboriginal |
| Miyakoshi, 2003 [106] | Universal screening at 24–27 wk; 1 h 50 g GCT ≥ 130 | JSOG | Retrospective; 1996–2000 | Keio University Hospital; data source not given, likely to be medical records | Japan | Japanese; 2651 | 1.8% |

Abbreviations: GCT, glucose challenge test; JSOG, Japanese Society of Obstetrics and Gynecology; NDDG, National Diabetes Data Group.
[a] Indicates that calendar time for participant enrollment was not provided; therefore, the publication date is substituted for the study time frame.
[b] Data source is provided for retrospective studies only.

of 2.6% in 1990 increasing to 3.8% in 2001, with significantly increasing rates of GDM in all major racial/ethnic groups except non-Hispanic whites [109]. The final study conducted in the United States used birth records of American Indian and white mothers in Montana and North Dakota for the years 1989 through 2000 [110]. In both states a statistically significant increase in prevalence of GDM was identified in whites, from 1.8% to 2.6% in Montana and from 1.6% to 3.2% in North Dakota [110]. In contrast, in the smaller population of American Indians within each state, a statistically significant increase in prevalence of GDM was reported for Montana (3.1%– 4.1%), but not North Dakota (3.8%–4.8%) [110].

The study conducted in Canada included over 100,000 perinatal records from 39 hospitals in Northern and Central Alberta and used NDDG criteria and universal screening throughout the study period [111]. The study reports a prevalence ranging between 2.2% and 2.8% between 1991 and 1997 with a nonsignificant test for linear trend for the duration of the study [111]. One of the three studies conducted in Australia is the only study to report a decrease in the prevalence of GDM over time [113]. The study was conducted in far North Queensland using a hospital database with 7567 entries [113]. Using ADIPS diagnostic criteria and universal screening with 78% to 85% of the population being screened throughout the study period, prevalence was 14.4% in 1992 and had dropped to 5.3% by 1996 [113]. Improvement in medical care and a dietary intervention were given as potential explanations for the decline in GDM during the study period [113]. A second study conducted in Australia included all deliveries in South Australia between 1988 and 1999 and reports an annual rate increase of 4.7% in the non-Aboriginal population, but not in the Aboriginal population (nonstatistically significant annual rate increase of 0.5%) [112]. Finally, using information on over 40,000 women attending Mercy Hospital for Women in Melbourne, Australia, a statistically significant increasing prevalence from 2.9% (1971–1980) to 8.8% (1991–1994) is reported [114].

## Discussion

In this study, the authors review studies published in the past 10 years that examine the prevalence and trends in the prevalence of GDM. In summary, the prevalence of GDM in a population is reflective of the prevalence of type 2 diabetes in that population; therefore, ethnic and racial populations that have a high prevalence of type 2 diabetes are at higher risk of GDM. In low-risk populations such as those found in Sweden, the prevalence in population-based studies is lower than 2% even when universal testing is offered [74–76], whereas studies in high-risk populations such as the Native American Cree, Northern Californian Hispanics, and Northern Californian Asians reported prevalence rates based on NDDG diagnostic criteria following universal screening ranging from 4.9% to 12.8% [64,68,70–72].

Table 5
Trends in the prevalence of GDM

| Author | Screening criteria | GDM criteria | Time frame[a] | Population/data source | Country | Ethnic group; n | Outcome |
|---|---|---|---|---|---|---|---|
| Dabelea, 2005 [107] | Universal screening at 24–28 wk; 1 h 50 g GCT $\geq$ 140; (96–98% screened) | NDDG | 1994–2002 | Kaiser Permanente of Colorado perinatal database, Denver metropolitan area | USA | NHW, Hispanic, AA, Asian; 36,403 | From 2.1% in 1994 to 4.1% in 2002; GDM prevalence increase was greater for minorities than whites |
| Thorpe, 2005 [108] | Screening and GDM criteria varied depending upon prenatal care received; however, universal screening has been practiced since the 1980s | | 1990–2001 | Residents of New York City with a singleton delivery; Birth certificate records from the New York City Department of Health and Mental Hygiene | USA | Diverse population; 1990; 125,663; 2001; 110,340 | From 2.6% in 1990 to 3.8% in 2001; GDM increased significantly in all major racial/ethnic groups except Non-Hispanic whites |
| Ferrara, 2004 [109] | Considered screened if a 1 h 50 g GCT (98.2% of those screened); 3 h 100 g OGTT (C&C); 2 h 75 g OGTT ($\geq$ 140); fasting glucose ($\geq$ 126; 2hr postprandial or random glucose measured ($\geq$ 200); 86.8% screened; GDM defined by above cutpoints or a hospital discharge diagnosis | | 1991–2000 | Northern California Kaiser Permanente Medical Care Program screened pregnancies; Gestational Diabetes Registry | USA | White, AA, Hispanic, Asian; 267,051 | From 5.1% in 1991 to 7.4% in 1997; leveled off through 2000 at 6.9% |
| Moum, 2004 [110] | Screening and GDM criteria varied depending upon prenatal care received | | 1989–2000 | American Indian and white mothers in Montana and North Dakota (ND); birth records | USA | Montana, 133,991; ND, 102,232 | Increasing rate of diabetes in pregnancy 1989 to 2000; 3.1 to 4.1%, Montana Indian; 1.8 to 2.6%, Montana white; 3.8 to 4.8%, ND Indian (NS); 1.6 to 3.2%, ND white |

| Study | Screening/Testing | Criteria | Years | Setting | Country | Population; N | Results |
|---|---|---|---|---|---|---|---|
| Xiong, 2001 [111] | Universal screening at 24–28 wk; 1 h 50 g GCT ≥ 140 | NDDG | 1991–1997 | 39 hospitals in Northern and Central Alberta; Perinatal Audit and Education Program records | Canada | Canadian; 111,563 | GDM prevalence ranged between 2.2–2.8% with a mean of 2.5% between 1991 and 1997; NS test for linear trend |
| Ishak, 2003 [112] | Unclear | ADIPS or WHO, 1999 | 1988–1999 | All deliveries in South Australia; Pregnancy Outcome Unit of the Department of Human Services | Australia | Aboriginal; 4,843 Non-Aboriginal; 225,168 | 4.3%, Aboriginal; 2.4%, Non-Aboriginal; Increasing trend in non-Aboriginal (annual rate increase of 4.7%), but not in Aboriginal population (0.5%) |
| Kim, 1999 [113] | Universal testing at 26–28 wk; 1 h 50 g GCT ≥ 140; (78%–85% screened) | ADIPS | 1992–1996 | Far North Queensland; Cairns Base Hospital database | Australia | Aboriginal, Torres Strait Islanders, Australian-born Caucasian, others; 7567 | 14.4%, 1992; 13.4%, 1993; 11.1%, 1994; 7.3%, 1995; 5.3%, 1996 |
| Beischer, 1996 [114] | Universal testing 3hr 50g OGTT; 1971 to 1980 at 30–34 wk (64.5% screened); 1981 and after at 30–34 wk (79.9% screened); GDM defined by a 1 h ≥ 162 and a 2 h ≥ 126 | JSOG; 1971 | 1971–1994 | Mercy Hospital for Women, Melbourne; either abstracted from medical records or a database | Australia | Not specified; 1971–1980; 27,111; 1991–1994; 16,820 | Of screened pregnancies from 2.9% in 1971–1980 to 8.8% in 1991–1994 ($X^2$ for trend, $P < .00001$) |

*Abbreviations:* AA, African American; JSOG, Japanese Society of Obstetrics and Gynecology; ND, North Dakota; NDDG, National Diabetes Data Group; NHW, non-Hispanic white; NS, not significant.

[a] All studies were retrospective.

Prevalence rates for GDM obtained from hospital-based studies similarly reflect the risk of type 2 diabetes in a population. A single hospital-based study in Australia using ADIPS diagnostic criteria and universal screening reports prevalences ranging from 3.0% in Anglo-Celtic women to 17.0% in Indian women [105]. Finally, of the eight studies published in the past 10 years that report on trends in the prevalence of GDM [107–114], one study reports a significant decline [113], one study reports no significant change [111], and six studies report an increase in the prevalence of GDM across most racial/ethnic groups studied [107–110,112,114].

Several factors influence the prevalence of GDM identified in a population and make it difficult to compare prevalences across populations. In the United States, the definition of GDM and screening policies concerning GDM have changed considerably in the past 20 years and still vary substantially. Despite four international conferences aimed at developing a consensus definition for GDM worldwide, the definition and screening criteria for GDM continue to vary, making it difficult to compare prevalences between countries. A critical change in the definition of GDM occurred at the 4th International Workshop conference on GDM in 1997, endorsed by the ADA, when it was largely agreed that the C&C criteria should replace the NDDG criteria, significantly lowering the accepted cutpoints and therefore raising the prevalence of GDM [61]. Finally, because GDM encompasses undiagnosed type 2 diabetes before pregnancy, the definition, screening strategies, and awareness of type 2 diabetes in a population ultimately influences the observed prevalence of GDM in a population. This is of particular importance during the past decade because the diagnostic criteria for diabetes and recommended screening practices have changed in the United States and internationally, namely the threshold for a fasting glucose level diagnostic of diabetes was lowered from 140 mg/dL to 126 mg/dL [115,116].

In addition to the varied definitions and screening policies for GDM and diabetes, there are several factors that make it difficult to compare GDM prevalence rates across populations and over time. Increased maternal age at delivery is a strong risk factor for GDM. Hence, a contributing factor to increased prevalence rates of GDM in a given population over time, or differences observed between populations, is increased maternal age at delivery. Because the authors are unable to age-standardize their prevalence rates across studies, they are unable to determine the impact of maternal age at delivery on prevalence rates across studies. However, increasing maternal age at delivery is one factor likely influencing the increasing prevalence of GDM in developed countries. Maternal age at delivery is also likely to vary and affect prevalence differences when comparing developed and undeveloped countries. Because the prevalence of GDM in a population reflects the prevalence of type 2 diabetes in a population, and certain racial and ethnic groups are at increased risk of type 2 diabetes, a second factor that may influence changes in prevalence overtime in a given population is a change in the racial/ethnic composition of that population. Although racial/ethnic group specific prevalences of GDM reflect the prevalence within a specific segment of the population, they may fail to reflect the broader public health impact of GDM as the overall population prevalence increases.

Changes in lifestyle including decreased physical activity and increased caloric consumption continue to fuel the obesity epidemic. Obesity, often accompanied by insulin resistance, is a strong risk factor for GDM and likely contributes to the increasing prevalence of GDM. The National Longitudinal Survey of Youth, a prospective cohort study of children aged 4 to 12 years performed between 1986 and 1998 in the United States, indicated that the prevalence of overweight children increased significantly and steadily throughout the study [117]. By the end of the study in 1998, obesity affected an estimated 21.5% of African American children, 21.8% of Hispanic children, and 12.3% of non-Hispanic white children [117]. In the 2003 to 2004 NHANES, 17.1% of individuals aged 2 to 19 years were overweight—more than triple the percent in 1980 [118]. In adults of childbearing age, the prevalence of obesity also continues to rise; in 18- to 29-year-olds, the prevalence of obesity rose from 7.1% in 1991 to 12.1% in 1998 in the Behavioral Risk Factor Surveillance System survey [119].

As obesity and diabetes increasingly affect young adults and women of childbearing age, understanding the public health impact of diabetes during pregnancy and its affect on infant health becomes important. Exposure to maternal diabetes later in pregnancy is associated with high birth weight, increased childhood and adult obesity, and increased risk of type 2 diabetes [41–48]. Therefore, the diabetic intrauterine environment may not only be a result of the obesity and diabetes epidemics, it may be partially responsible and currently fueling the epidemics. Moreover, because both obesity and diabetes disproportionately affect minority women including minority women of childbearing age [8,16], if the intrauterine environment is contributing to the epidemics, it perpetuates and widens health disparities between racial and ethnic groups.

The population health impact of GDM is not limited to exposed offspring, but affects maternal health as well. Once diagnosed with GDM, a woman has a substantial chance of developing type 2 diabetes following delivery, with some studies reporting a 5-year cumulative incidence rate of over 50% [120]. Moreover, because childbearing women are young, women who have GDM who develop overt diabetes acquire it at a young age, substantially increasing their lifetime risk of developing complications from diabetes. The Diabetes Prevention Program was one of several clinical trials that indicated that either through diet and exercise, or with the aid of a pharmacologic agent, it is possible to lower the incidence or delay the onset of diabetes among individuals at high risk of the disease [121–124]. Women who have GDM, because of their high diabetes risk and young age, are ideally suited to be targeted for lifestyle or pharmacologic interventions to delay or prevent the onset of overt diabetes [121–124]. Moreover, because women who have GDM are of childbearing age, preventing or delaying the onset of overt diabetes not only improves the woman's health, but also protects future offspring from the harmful effects of elevated glucose levels in pregnancy [125,126].

In summary, diabetes during pregnancy is a common and increasing complication of pregnancy that differentially affects racial and ethnic minority populations dependent upon their underlying risk of diabetes. Hence, an important public health priority, consistent with reducing health disparities between racial and ethnic groups, is prevention of diabetes, starting with maternal health pre- and postconception.

## References

[1] Burke JP, Williams K, Gaskill SP, et al. Rapid rise in the incidence of type 2 diabetes from 1987 to 1996: results from the San Antonio Heart Study. Arch Intern Med 1999; 159:1450–6.

[2] Dabelea D, Pettitt DJ, Jones KL, et al. Type 2 diabetes mellitus in minority children and adolescents. An emerging problem. Endocrinol Metab Clin North Am 1999;28:709–29, [viii].

[3] Fagot-Campagna A, Pettitt DJ, Engelgau MM, et al. Type 2 diabetes among North American children and adolescents: an epidemiologic review and a public health perspective. J Pediatr 2000;136:664–72.

[4] Fagot-Campagna A, Saaddine JB, Flegal KM, et al. Diabetes, impaired fasting glucose, and elevated HbA1c in U.S. adolescents: the Third National Health and Nutrition Examination Survey. Diabetes Care 2001;24:834–7.

[5] Harris MI, Flegal KM, Cowie CC, et al. Prevalence of diabetes, impaired fasting glucose, and impaired glucose tolerance in U.S. adults. The Third National Health and Nutrition Examination Survey, 1988–1994. Diabetes Care 1998;21:518–24.

[6] Rosenbloom AL, Joe JR, Young RS, et al. Emerging epidemic of type 2 diabetes in youth. Diabetes Care 1999;22:345–54.

[7] Cowie CC, Rust KF, Byrd-Holt DD, et al. Prevalence of diabetes and impaired fasting glucose in adults in the U.S. population: National Health and Nutrition Examination Survey 1999-2002. Diabetes Care 2006;29:1263–8.

[8] Narayan KM, Boyle JP, Thompson TJ, et al. Lifetime risk for diabetes mellitus in the United States. JAMA 2003;290:1884–90.

[9] Wild S, Roglic G, Green A, et al. Global prevalence of diabetes: estimates for the year 2000 and projections for 2030. Diabetes Care 2004;27:1047–53.

[10] Pan XR, Yang WY, Li GW, et al. Prevalence of diabetes and its risk factors in China, 1994. National Diabetes Prevention and Control Cooperative Group. Diabetes Care 1997;20: 1664–9.

[11] Ramachandran A, Snehalatha C, Kapur A, et al. High prevalence of diabetes and impaired glucose tolerance in India: National Urban Diabetes Survey. Diabetologia 2001;44: 1094–101.

[12] World Health Organization. Obesity: preventing and manageing the global epidemic. Geneva (Switzerland): World Health Organization; 2000 [World Health Organization Technical Support Series No. 894].

[13] Wang Y. Cross-national comparison of childhood obesity: the epidemic and the relationship between obesity and socioeconomic status. Int J Epidemiol 2001;30:1129–36.

[14] Centers for Disease Control. Update: prevalence of overweight among children, adolescents, and adults—United States, 1988-1994. MMWR Morb Mortal Wkly Rep 1997;46: 198–202.

[15] Troiano RP, Flegal KM, Kuczmarski RJ, et al. Overweight prevalence and trends for children and adolescents. The National Health and Nutrition Examination Surveys, 1963 to 1991. Arch Pediatr Adolesc Med 1995;149:1085–91.

[16] Flegal KM, Carroll MD, Ogden CL, et al. Prevalence and trends in obesity among US adults, 1999-2000. JAMA 2002;288:1723–7.

[17] Ogden CL, Flegal KM, Carroll MD, et al. Prevalence and trends in overweight among US children and adolescents, 1999–2000. JAMA 2002;288:1728–32.

[18] Hedley AA, Ogden CL, Johnson CL, et al. Prevalence of overweight and obesity among US children, adolescents, and adults, 1999-2002. JAMA 2004;291:2847–50.

[19] Barker DJ. Fetal origins of coronary heart disease. BMJ 1995;311:171–4.

[20] Lucas A. Programming by early nutrition in man. In: Bock GR, Whelan J, editors. The childhood environment and adult disease. Chichester (UK): John Wiley and Sons; 1991. p. 38–55.

[21] Ravelli AC, van der Meulen JH, Osmond C, et al. Obesity at the age of 50 y in men and women exposed to famine prenatally. Am J Clin Nutr 1999;70:811–6.

[22] Ravelli GP, Stein ZA, Susser MW. Obesity in young men after famine exposure in utero and early infancy. N Engl J Med 1976;295:349–53.

[23] Hales CN, Barker DJ, Clark PM, et al. Fetal and infant growth and impaired glucose tolerance at age 64. BMJ 1991;303:1019–22.

[24] Hales CN, Barker DJ. Type 2 (non-insulin-dependent) diabetes mellitus: the thrifty phenotype hypothesis. Diabetologia 1992;35:595–601.

[25] Valdez R, Athens MA, Thompson GH, et al. Birthweight and adult health outcomes in a biethnic population in the USA. Diabetologia 1994;37:624–31.

[26] McCance DR, Pettitt DJ, Hanson RL, et al. Birth weight and non-insulin dependent diabetes: thrifty genotype, thrifty phenotype, or surviving small baby genotype? BMJ 1994; 308:942–5.

[27] Rich-Edwards JW, Colditz GA, Stampfer MJ, et al. Birthweight and the risk for type 2 diabetes mellitus in adult women. Ann Intern Med 1999;130:278–84.

[28] Robinson S, Walton RJ, Clark PM, et al. The relation of fetal growth to plasma glucose in young men. Diabetologia 1992;35:444–6.

[29] Curhan GC, Chertow GM, Willett WC, et al. Birth weight and adult hypertension and obesity in women. Circulation 1996;94:1310–5.

[30] Curhan GC, Willett WC, Rimm EB, et al. Birth weight and adult hypertension, diabetes mellitus, and obesity in US men. Circulation 1996;94:3246–50.

[31] Barker DJ, Osmond C, Golding J, et al. Growth in utero, blood pressure in childhood and adult life, and mortality from cardiovascular disease. BMJ 1989;298: 564–7.

[32] Barker DJ, Bull AR, Osmond C, et al. Fetal and placental size and risk of hypertension in adult life. BMJ 1990;301:259–62.

[33] Law CM, de Swiet M, Osmond C, et al. Initiation of hypertension in utero and its amplification throughout adult life. BMJ 1993;306:24–7.

[34] Rich-Edwards JW, Stampfer MJ, Manson JE, et al. Birth weight and risk of cardiovascular disease in a cohort of women followed up since 1976. BMJ 1997;315:396–400.

[35] Osmond C, Barker DJ, Winter PD, et al. Early growth and death from cardiovascular disease in women. BMJ 1993;307:1519–24.

[36] Fall CH, Vijayakumar M, Barker DJ, et al. Weight in infancy and prevalence of coronary heart disease in adult life. BMJ 1995;310:17–9.

[37] Berkowitz GS, Lapinski RH, Wein R, et al. Race/ethnicity and other risk factors for gestational diabetes. Am J Epidemiol 1992;135:965–73.

[38] Solomon CG, Willett WC, Carey VJ, et al. A prospective study of pregravid determinants of gestational diabetes mellitus. JAMA 1997;278:1078–83.

[39] Dornhorst A, Paterson CM, Nicholls JS, et al. High prevalence of gestational diabetes in women from ethnic minority groups. Diabet Med 1992;9:820–5.

[40] Zhang S, Folsom AR, Flack JM, et al. Body fat distribution before pregnancy and gestational diabetes: findings from coronary artery risk development in young adults (CARDIA) study. BMJ 1995;311:1139–40.

[41] Freinkel N. Banting lecture 1980. Of pregnancy and progeny. Diabetes 1980;29:1023–35.

[42] Dabelea D, Hanson RL, Bennett PH, et al. Increasing prevalence of type II diabetes in American Indian children. Diabetologia 1998;41:904–10.

[43] Silverman BL, Rizzo T, Green OC, et al. Long-term prospective evaluation of offspring of diabetic mothers. Diabetes 1991;40(Suppl 2):121–5.

[44] O'Sullivan JB, Gellis SS, Dandrow RV, et al. The potential diabetic and her treatment in pregnancy. Obstet Gynecol 1966;27:683–9.

[45] Dabelea D, Hanson RL, Lindsay RS, et al. Intrauterine exposure to diabetes conveys risks for type 2 diabetes and obesity: a study of discordant sibships. Diabetes 2000;49:2208–11.

[46] Pettitt DJ, Knowler WC, Baird HR, et al. Gestational diabetes: infant and maternal complications of pregnancy in relation to third-trimester glucose tolerance in the Pima Indians. Diabetes Care 1980;3:458–64.

[47] Pettitt DJ, Knowler WC, Bennett PH, et al. Obesity in offspring of diabetic Pima Indian women despite normal birth weight. Diabetes Care 1987;10:76–80.

[48] Pettitt DJ, Knowler WC. Long-term effects of the intrauterine environment, birth weight, and breast-feeding in Pima Indians. Diabetes Care 1998;21(Suppl 2):B138–41.

[49] Pettitt DJ, Aleck KA, Baird HR, et al. Congenital susceptibility to NIDDM. Role of intrauterine environment. Diabetes 1988;37:622–8.

[50] Hanson RL, Elston RC, Pettitt DJ, et al. Segregation analysis of non-insulin-dependent diabetes mellitus in Pima Indians: evidence for a major-gene effect. Am J Hum Genet 1995;57:160–70.

[51] Report of a WHO Study Group. Diabetes mellitus: Report of a WHO Study Group. Geneva (Switzerland): World Health Organization; 1985. Technical Report Series 727. 727, 1–113.

[52] Lind T, Phillips PR. Influence of pregnancy on the 75-g OGTT. A prospective multicenter study. The Diabetic Pregnancy Study Group of the European Association for the Study of Diabetes. Diabetes 1991;40(Suppl 2):8–13.

[53] ACOG technical bulletin. Diabetes and pregnancy. Number 200—December 1994 (replaces No. 92, May 1986). Committee on Technical Bulletins of the American College of Obstetricians and Gynecologists. Int J Gynaecol Obstet 1995;48:331–9.

[54] Hoffman L, Nolan C, Wilson JD, et al. Gestational diabetes mellitus—management guidelines. The Australasian Diabetes in Pregnancy Society. Med J Aust 1998;169:93–7.

[55] O'Sullivan JB, Mahan C. Criteria for the oral glucose tolerance test in pregnancy. Diabetes 1964;13:278–85.

[56] Sugawa T. Report from a committee on nutritional and metabolic problems. Nippon Sanka Fujinka Gakkai Zasshi 1984;36:2055–8.

[57] Carpenter MW, Coustan DR. Criteria for screening tests for gestational diabetes. Am J Obstet Gynecol 1982;144:768–73.

[58] National Diabetes Data Group. Classification and diagnosis of diabetes mellitus and other categories of glucose intolerance. National Diabetes Data Group. Diabetes 1979;28:1039–57.

[59] American Diabetes Association. American Diabetes Association clinical practice recommendations 2001. Diabetes Care 2001;24(Suppl 1): S1–133.

[60] ACOG Practice Bulletin. Clinical management guidelines for obstetrician-gynecologists. Number 30, September 2001 (replaces Technical Bulletin Number 200, December 1994). Gestational diabetes. Obstet Gynecol 2001;98:525–38.

[61] Metzger BE, Coustan DR. Summary and recommendations of the Fourth International Workshop-Conference on Gestational Diabetes Mellitus. The Organizing Committee. Diabetes Care 1998;21(Suppl 2):B161–7.

[62] Rosenberg TJ, Garbers S, Lipkind H, et al. Maternal obesity and diabetes as risk factors for adverse pregnancy outcomes: differences among 4 racial/ethnic groups. Am J Public Health 2005;95:1545–51.

[63] Williams MA, Emanuel I, Kimpo C, et al. A population-based cohort study of the relation between maternal birthweight and risk of gestational diabetes mellitus in four racial/ethnic groups. Paediatr Perinat Epidemiol 1999;13:452–65.

[64] Godwin M, Muirhead M, Huynh J, et al. Prevalence of gestational diabetes mellitus among Swampy Cree women in Moose Factory, James Bay. CMAJ 1999;160:1299–302.

[65] Janghorbani M, Stenhouse E, Jones RB, et al. Gestational diabetes mellitus in Plymouth, U.K.: prevalence, seasonal variation and associated factors. J Reprod Med 2006;51:128–34.

[66] Weijers RN, Bekedam DJ, Oosting H. The prevalence of type 2 diabetes and gestational diabetes mellitus in an inner city multi-ethnic population. Eur J Epidemiol 1998;14: 693–9.

[67] Stone CA, McLachlan KA, Halliday JL, et al. Gestational diabetes in Victoria in 1996: incidence, risk factors and outcomes. Med J Aust 2002;177:486–91.

[68] Ferrara A, Hedderson MM, Quesenberry CP, et al. Prevalence of gestational diabetes mellitus detected by the national diabetes data group or the carpenter and coustan plasma glucose thresholds. Diabetes Care 2002;25:1625–30.

[69] Kieffer EC, Carman WJ, Gillespie BW, et al. Obesity and gestational diabetes among African-American women and Latinas in Detroit: implications for disparities in women's health. J Am Med Womens Assoc 2001;56:181–7, 196.

[70] Rodrigues S, Robinson E, Gray-Donald K. Prevalence of gestational diabetes mellitus among James Bay Cree women in northern Quebec. CMAJ 1999;160:1293–7.

[71] Rodrigues S, Robinson EJ, Ghezzo H, et al. Interaction of body weight and ethnicity on risk of gestational diabetes mellitus. Am J Clin Nutr 1999;70:1083–9.

[72] Harris SB, Caulfield LE, Sugamori ME, et al. The epidemiology of diabetes in pregnant Native Canadians. A risk profile. Diabetes Care 1997;20:1422–5.

[73] Schmidt MI, Duncan BB, Reichelt AJ, et al. Gestational diabetes mellitus diagnosed with a 2-h 75-g oral glucose tolerance test and adverse pregnancy outcomes. Diabetes Care 2001; 24:1151–5.

[74] Ostlund I, Hanson U. Occurrence of gestational diabetes mellitus and the value of different screening indicators for the oral glucose tolerance test. Acta Obstet Gynecol Scand 2003;82: 103–8.

[75] Ostlund I, Hanson U. Repeated random blood glucose measurements as universal screening test for gestational diabetes mellitus. Acta Obstet Gynecol Scand 2004;83:46–51.

[76] Aberg AE, Jonsson EK, Eskilsson I, et al. Predictive factors of developing diabetes mellitus in women with gestational diabetes. Acta Obstet Gynecol Scand 2002;81:11–6.

[77] Jensen DM, Molsted-Pedersen L, Beck-Nielsen H, et al. Screening for gestational diabetes mellitus by a model based on risk indicators: a prospective study. Am J Obstet Gynecol 2003;189:1383–8.

[78] Kvetny J, Poulsen HF, Damgaard DW. Results from screening for gestational diabetes mellitus in a Danish county. Dan Med Bull 1999;46:57–9.

[79] Di Cianni G, Benzi L, Casadidio I, et al. Screening of gestational diabetes in Tuscany: results in 2000 cases. Ann Ist Super Sanita 1997;33:389–91.

[80] Murgia C, Berria R, Minerba L, et al. Gestational diabetes mellitus in Sardinia: results from an early, universal screening procedure. Diabetes Care 2006;29:1713–4.

[81] Erem C, Cihanyurdu N, Deger O, et al. Screening for gestational diabetes mellitus in northeastern Turkey (Trabzon City). Eur J Epidemiol 2003;18:39–43.

[82] Keshavarz M, Cheung NW, Babaee GR, et al. Gestational diabetes in Iran: incidence, risk factors and pregnancy outcomes. Diabetes Res Clin Pract 2005;69:279–86.

[83] Hadaegh F, Tohidi M, Harati H, et al. Prevalence of gestational diabetes mellitus in southern Iran (Bandar Abbas City). Endocr Pract 2005;11:313–8.

[84] Al Mahroos S, Nagalla DS, Yousif W, et al. A population-based screening for gestational diabetes mellitus in non-diabetic women in Bahrain. Ann Saudi Med 2005;25:129–33.

[85] Seyoum B, Kiros K, Haileselase T, et al. Prevalence of gestational diabetes mellitus in rural pregnant mothers in northern Ethiopia. Diabetes Res Clin Pract 1999;46:247–51.

[86] Zargar AH, Sheikh MI, Bashir MI, et al. Prevalence of gestational diabetes mellitus in Kashmiri women from the Indian subcontinent. Diabetes Res Clin Pract 2004;66: 139–45.

[87] Yang X, Hsu-Hage B, Zhang H, et al. Gestational diabetes mellitus in women of single gravidity in Tianjin City, China. Diabetes Care 2002;25:847–51.

[88] Maegawa Y, Sugiyama T, Kusaka H, et al. Screening tests for gestational diabetes in Japan in the 1st and 2nd trimester of pregnancy. Diabetes Res Clin Pract 2003;62:47–53.

[89] Santos-Ayarzagoitia M, Salinas-Martinez AM, Villarreal-Perez JZ. Gestational diabetes: validity of ADA and WHO diagnostic criteria using NDDG as the reference test. Diabetes Res Clin Pract 2006;74(3):322–8.

[90] Ricart W, Lopez J, Mozas J, et al. Potential impact of American Diabetes Association (2000) criteria for diagnosis of gestational diabetes mellitus in Spain. Diabetologia 2005; 48:1135–41.

[91] Corrado F, Stella NC, Mancuso A, et al. Screening for gestational diabetes in Sicily. J Reprod Med 1999;44:875–8.

[92] Yogev Y, Langer O, Xenakis EM, et al. Glucose screening in Mexican-American women. Obstet Gynecol 2004;103:1241–5.

[93] Stamilio DM, Olsen T, Ratcliffe S, et al. False-positive 1-hour glucose challenge test and adverse perinatal outcomes. Obstet Gynecol 2004;103:148–56.

[94] Danilenko-Dixon DR, Van Winter JT, Nelson RL, et al. Universal versus selective gestational diabetes screening: application of 1997 American Diabetes Association recommendations. Am J Obstet Gynecol 1999;181:798–802.

[95] Dyck R, Klomp H, Tan LK, et al. A comparison of rates, risk factors, and outcomes of gestational diabetes between aboriginal and non-aboriginal women in the Saskatoon health district. Diabetes Care 2002;25:487–93.

[96] Jimenez-Moleon JJ, Bueno-Cavanillas A, Luna-Del-Castillo JD, et al. Prevalence of gestational diabetes mellitus: variations related to screening strategy used. Eur J Endocrinol 2002;146:831–7.

[97] Bartha JL, Martinez-Del-Fresno P, Comino-Delgado R. Gestational diabetes mellitus diagnosed during early pregnancy. Am J Obstet Gynecol 2000;182:346–50.

[98] Di Cianni G, Volpe L, Lencioni C, et al. Prevalence and risk factors for gestational diabetes assessed by universal screening. Diabetes Res Clin Pract 2003;62:131–7.

[99] Yalcin HR, Zorlu CG. Threshold value of glucose screening tests in pregnancy: could it be standardized for every population? Am J Perinatol 1996;13:317–20.

[100] Larijani B, Hossein-nezhad A, Rizvi SW, et al. Cost analysis of different screening strategies for gestational diabetes mellitus. Endocr Pract 2003;9:504–9.

[101] Hassan A. Screening of pregnant women for gestational diabetes mellitus. J Ayub Med Coll Abbottabad 2005;17:54–8.

[102] Seshiah V, Balaji V, Balaji MS, et al. Gestational diabetes mellitus in India. J Assoc Physicians India 2004;52:707–11.

[103] Wagaarachchi PT, Fernando L, Premachadra P, et al. Screening based on risk factors for gestational diabetes in an Asian population. J Obstet Gynaecol 2001;21:32–4.

[104] Davey RX, Hamblin PS. Selective versus universal screening for gestational diabetes mellitus: an evaluation of predictive risk factors. Med J Aust 2001;174:118–21.

[105] Yue DK, Molyneaux LM, Ross GP, et al. Why does ethnicity affect prevalence of gestational diabetes? The underwater volcano theory. Diabet Med 1996;13:748–52.

[106] Miyakoshi K, Tanaka M, Ueno K, et al. Cutoff value of 1 h, 50 g glucose challenge test for screening of gestational diabetes mellitus in a Japanese population. Diabetes Res Clin Pract 2003;60:63–7.

[107] Dabelea D, Snell-Bergeon JK, Hartsfield CL, et al. Increasing prevalence of gestational diabetes mellitus (GDM) over time and by birth cohort: Kaiser Permanente of Colorado GDM Screening Program. Diabetes Care 2005;28:579–84.

[108] Thorpe LE, Berger D, Ellis JA, et al. Trends and racial/ethnic disparities in gestational diabetes among pregnant women in New York City, 1990-2001. Am J Public Health 2005;95: 1536–9.

[109] Ferrara A, Kahn HS, Quesenberry CP, et al. An increase in the incidence of gestational diabetes mellitus: Northern California, 1991–2000. Obstet Gynecol 2004;103:526–33.

[110] Moum KR, Holzman GS, Harwell TS, et al. Increasing rate of diabetes in pregnancy among American Indian and white mothers in Montana and North Dakota, 1989–2000. Matern Child Health J 2004;8:71–6.

[111] Xiong X, Saunders LD, Wang FL, et al. Gestational diabetes mellitus: prevalence, risk factors, maternal and infant outcomes. Int J Gynaecol Obstet 2001;75:221–8.

[112] Ishak M, Petocz P. Gestational diabetes among Aboriginal Australians: prevalence, time trend, and comparisons with non-Aboriginal Australians. Ethn Dis 2003;13:55–60.

[113] Kim S, Humphrey MD. Decrease in incidence of gestational diabetes mellitus in Far North Queensland between 1992 and 1996. Aust N Z J Obstet Gynaecol 1999;39:40–3.

[114] Beischer NA, Wein P, Sheedy MT, et al. Identification and treatment of women with hyperglycaemia diagnosed during pregnancy can significantly reduce perinatal mortality rates. Aust N Z J Obstet Gynaecol 1996;36:239–47.

[115] Report of the Expert Committee on the diagnosis and classification of diabetes mellitus. Diabetes Care 1997;20:1183–97.

[116] Report of a WHO Consultation. Definition, Diagnosis and Classification of Diabetes Mellitus and its Complications. Part 1: Diagnosis and Classification of Diabetes Mellitus. In: Alwan A, King H. Geneva (Switzerland): World Health Organization. Department of Noncommunicable Disease Surveillance; 1999. p. 1–59.

[117] Strauss RS, Pollack HA. Epidemic increase in childhood overweight, 1986-1998. JAMA 2001;286:2845–8.

[118] Ogden CL, Carroll MD, Curtin LR, et al. Prevalence of overweight and obesity in the United States, 1999-2004. JAMA 2006;295:1549–55.

[119] Mokdad AH, Serdula MK, Dietz WH, et al. The spread of the obesity epidemic in the United States, 1991-1998. JAMA 1999;282:1519–22.

[120] Kim C, Newton KM, Knopp RH. Gestational diabetes and the incidence of type 2 diabetes: a systematic review. Diabetes Care 2002;25:1862–8.

[121] Chiasson JL, Josse RG, Gomis R, et al. Acarbose for prevention of type 2 diabetes mellitus: the STOP-NIDDM randomised trial. Lancet 2002;359:2072–7.

[122] Knowler WC, Barrett-Connor E, Fowler SE, et al. Reduction in the incidence of type 2 diabetes with lifestyle intervention or metformin. N Engl J Med 2002;346:393–403.

[123] Pan XR, Li GW, Hu YH, et al. Effects of diet and exercise in preventing NIDDM in people with impaired glucose tolerance. The Da Qing IGT and Diabetes Study. Diabetes Care 1997;20:537–44.

[124] Tuomilehto J, Lindstrom J, Eriksson JG, et al. Prevention of type 2 diabetes mellitus by changes in lifestyle among subjects with impaired glucose tolerance. N Engl J Med 2001; 344:1343–50.

[125] Dabelea D, Knowler WC, Pettitt DJ. Effect of diabetes in pregnancy on offspring: follow-up research in the Pima Indians. J Matern Fetal Med 2000;9:83–8.

[126] Dabelea D, Pettitt DJ. Intrauterine diabetic environment confers risks for type 2 diabetes mellitus and obesity in the offspring, in addition to genetic susceptibility. J Pediatr Endocrinol Metab 2001;14:1085–91.

ELSEVIER
SAUNDERS

Obstet Gynecol Clin N Am
34 (2007) 201–212

OBSTETRICS AND
GYNECOLOGY
CLINICS
OF NORTH AMERICA

# In Utero Exposure to Maternal Obesity and Diabetes: Animal Models That Identify and Characterize Implications for Future Health

Peter W. Nathanielsz, MD, PhD, ScD, FRCOG[a],*,
Lucilla Poston, PhD, FRCOG[b], Paul D. Taylor, PhD[b]

[a]Department of Obstetrics & Gynecology, Center for Pregnancy and Newborn Research,
The University of Texas of Health Science Center, 7703 Floyd Curl Drive,
MSC 7836, San Antonio, TX 78229, USA
[b]Maternal & Fetal Unit, Department of Women's Health, Division of Reproduction
and Endocrinology, King's College London, 10th Floor, North Wing,
St. Thomas' Hospital, London SE1, 7EH, UK

The developed and developing worlds are experiencing an epidemic of obesity and associated predisposition to diabetes. This epidemic places a major drain on health care resources. In the United States, estimates suggest that one third of adult women are clinically obese [1]. This increased incidence of obesity and diabetes includes women of child-bearing age [2–4]. It is now clear that maternal obesity and gestational diabetes have major adverse effects on the developing fetus that lead to increased neonatal morbidity and mortality, as discussed elsewhere in this issue. Obesity in pregnancy and gestational diabetes represent a special problem, not only as a result of their immediate adverse effects on maternal health and pregnancy outcome, but also because of growing evidence for their persistent and deleterious effects on the developing child.

Recent human epidemiologic observations and experimental studies in rodents and sheep [5–10] show that the nutrient environment in which the fetus and neonate develop can alter the trajectory of development of multiple organ systems in ways that permanently impair their function and predispose the offspring to chronic diseases that only emerge in later life. The persistent effects of a suboptimal fetal and neonatal development have been called

NICHD HD 21350.
* Corresponding author.
  E-mail address: nathanielsz@uthscsa.edu (P.W. Nathanielsz).

0889-8545/07/$ - see front matter © 2007 Elsevier Inc. All rights reserved.
doi:10.1016/j.ogc.2007.03.006

*developmental programming.* Developmental programming can be defined as *the response to a specific challenge to the mammalian organism during a critical developmental time window that alters the trajectory of development qualitatively and/or quantitatively with resulting persistent effects on phenotype.* The fundamental principles of developmental programming are laid out in Box 1.

The nutritional environment experienced during fetal and early postnatal life is proposed to affect susceptibility to the development of cardiovascular disease and glucose intolerance later in life [11]. Numerous human cohort studies have demonstrated an association of low weight at birth with facets of metabolic syndrome, including hypertension, glucose intolerance, and obesity [12–14]. Catch-up growth in early postnatal life or childhood seems to further increase the risk of developing these predisposing conditions, which have strong associations with cardiovascular disease [15–18].

## Maternal obesity and consequences for the developing child

In view of the rising birth weight in developed countries, the prevalence of obesity in pregnancy, and the association with gestational diabetes, there is increasing interest in the potentially detrimental influence of a maternal hyper-nutritional status and associated raised birth weight on the risk of disease in the child [19–23]. Though the link between obesity, gestational diabetes and heavier weight at birth is recognized, it is increasingly clear that obesity per se may also contribute. Indeed weight gain between first and second pregnancies has recently been recognized as a factor that increases the risk of the second baby being large for gestational age, even amongst women who are not clinically obese [4]. Prolonged effects of obesity in the mother have also been implicated from cohort studies that document prepregnancy body mass index as a strong and independent determinant of their child becoming overweight [24]. Several studies show a U- or J-shaped relationship between birth weight and later insulin resistance and obesity [25–27]. Children of obese women who are diabetic in pregnancy are themselves more likely to develop insulin resistance in later life and to become overweight [28,29]. While this predisposition may represent in part a genetically inherited disorder, studies among the Pima Arizonian Indians of siblings, who were discordant for maternal diabetes, strongly suggest an acquired diabetic trait [30,31]. Others have reported increased risk of metabolic syndrome (raised blood pressure, increased adiposity, insulin resistance) not only among children who were born large for gestational age to mothers who had gestational diabetes but also amongst those overweight at birth whose mothers were nondiabetic [32].

## Mechanisms by which maternal obesity and gestational diabetes produce their unwanted effects on lifetime offspring health

Maternal hyperglycaemia is usually thought of as the predominant driving influence in the tendency of obese and diabetic women to have large for

**Box 1. Ten principles of developmental programming**

1. During development, there are **critical periods of vulnerability** to suboptimal conditions. Vulnerable periods occur at different times for different tissues. Cells dividing rapidly are at greatest risk. Factors that increase risk include:
   Too much of a normal chemical such as a hormone, critical nutrient, or vitamin
   Deficiency of a normal chemical such as a hormone, critical nutrient, or vitamin
   Abnormal chemicals such as alcohol or nicotine
   Abnormal physical forces, such as high blood pressure
2. Programming has **permanent effects** that alter responses in later life and can modify susceptibility to disease.
3. Fetal development is fetal physical **activity–dependent.** Normal development is dependent on continuing normal activity. Each phase of development provides the required conditions for subsequent development.
4. Programming may involve structural changes in important organs.
   The absolute numbers of cells in the organ may increase or decrease.
   The relative proportions and distribution of different types of cells within the organ may be unbalanced.
   The normal blood supply to the organ may be compromised.
   Too many or too few hormone receptors may form with a resultant resetting of feedback and other control mechanisms.
5. The **placenta** is likely to play a key role in some forms of programming.
6. **Compensation carries a price.** In an unfavorable environment, the developing baby makes attempts to compensate for deficiencies. Following compensation, birth weight may be normal or only slightly decreased. However, the compensatory effort carries a price.
7. Attempts made after birth to reverse the consequences of programming may have their own unwanted consequences. When postnatal conditions prove to be other than those for which the fetus prepared, problems may arise.
8. **Fetal cellular mechanisms often differ from adult processes.** Fetuses react differently to suboptimal conditions than do newborn babies or adults.
9. The **effects of programming may pass across generations** by mechanisms that do not necessarily involve changes in the genes.
10. Programming often has different effects in males and females.

gestational age babies, but studies in diabetic pregnancies suggest that pre-pregnancy maternal body composition and hitherto unrecognized factors may have equally important influences [33]. Obesity and maternal diabetes are associated with abnormalities in maternal lipid and amino acid metabo-lism in addition to altered glucose metabolism. Large birth weight can un-doubtedly be associated with a higher adult body mass index but in association with increased muscle mass rather than fat mass [34]. Contempo-rary studies are now addressing this by detailed measurement of body com-position in the child in relation to maternal obesity and gestational diabetes. Thus Catalano and colleagues [21,22] have shown that children of mothers who have gestational diabetes have a greater neonatal fat mass than children of the same birth weight whose mothers did not have diabetes in pregnancy. Importantly the same group have now reported that infants of obese nondi-abetic mothers are likely to be fatter than those of lean mothers, even when the birth weights are little different [35]. The association between maternal obesity, with or without gestational diabetes, and the body composition of the developing child through to adulthood requires better definition and, al-though currently underway in some large cohorts, will take many years to elucidate. Prospective investigation of human cohorts, although of enormous value in determining associations between maternal nutritional status and offspring outcome are complex, expensive, and confounded by the influence of uncontrollable variables of genetic and environmental origin. There is a need for information at the level of gene expression, gene product forma-tion, cell and tissue activity, as well as determination of whole body pheno-type. Studies in appropriate animal models are needed to speed our understanding of the adverse consequences of maternal obesity and diabetes on offspring. Information from animal studies is indispensable to pave the way to identification of markers of problems as well as better prevention and clinical management.

## Experimental animal models

The use of models in experimental animals has provided a supplementary approach to human epidemiologic and clinical studies. Data from animal models of developmental programming have been informative in understanding exposures, mechanisms, and outcomes. It seems that the de-veloping cardiovascular system and pathways of glucose and fat metabolism are particularly prone to perturbation in the presence of maternal nutri-tional imbalance and other alterations in the maternal environment and phenotype. To date, experimental studies on the developmental programming of obesity and diabetes in offspring have generally focused on maternal and fetal undernutrition, rather than the effects of maternal overnutrition, obesity, and gestational diabetes.

The various animal models that have been studied in relation to maternal overnutrition during pregnancy and lactation have been reviewed [5–7]. The vast majority of studies have been conducted in rodents and sheep. As shown in one of the earliest studies on developmental programming due to overnutrition during development, effects are sex-of-offspring–dependent. Thus overfeeding neonatal baboons before weaning resulted in fat cell hypertrophy in female offspring only [36]. This latter study highlights two important principles of developmental programming. First it shows the importance of studying the whole developmental period. One of the basic principles of developmental programming is that there are critical windows of vulnerability (see Box 1, principle 1), and these windows may be prenatal or postnatal. It is also important to consider differential timing of the relative stages of development in different animal species when extrapolating findings from animal studies to human development. The extensive studies in rodents during the neonatal period must be interpreted in the light of the precocial prenatal development of many systems in humans and other mammals. Thus, evidence obtained by alterations in nutrition in the suckling period in the altricial rat is likely to relate to changes during fetal development in precocial mammals. Secondly, it is important to look for gender-specific effects in outcomes.

Evidence from cross-fostering studies have demonstrated that overfeeding in the neonatal period can lead to offspring adiposity associated with hyperleptinemia and hypertension When litter size is reduced in rodents during the preweaning period, thereby leading to over nutrition, offspring are hyperphagic and obese [37]. The hyperglycemia that occurs in rats that exhibit gestational diabetes has been shown to program adult obesity and changes in the hypothalamic appetite regulatory centers (see later discussion).

## Altered regulation of appetite and physical activity

Obesity results from an imbalance of energy intake and energy use—metabolic rate and physical activity. The hypothalamic centers that regulate the orexigenic drive to eat and the balancing anorexigenic drive that represents satiety develop in late gestation in primates, although the development continues into the postnatal period [38,39]. In rodents, development is mostly postnatal and hence easier to manipulate experimentally. In the arcuate nucleus area of the hypothalamus, neuropeptide Y and agouti-related protein neurons are the major site of the orexigenic drive, while proopiomelanocortin and cocaine and amphetamineregulated transcript-secreting neurons provide the anorexigenic drive leptin produced by adipose tissue, feeds back on these areas to decrease appetite [38].

Overfeeding of neonatal rat pups produced by reducing litter size to four pups results in offspring hyperphagia and adiposity [40], hyperleptinemia, hyperinsulinaemia, and resistance to leptin feedback on the arcuate nucleus [41]. The increase in feeding in response to neuropeptide Y injection into the lateral ventricle of the brain is exaggerated in 6-month-old offspring of mothers who were fed a high-fat diet [42]. Weanling pups of dams who were fed a high-fat diet show up-regulation of appetite stimulatory galanin and orexin mRNA expression in the paraventricular nucleus and lateral hypothalamus, respectively [43]. However, the pups in both studies, in contrast to other reports of maternal fat feeding, were born smaller than controls, and the response may represent a compensatory "catch-up" response. In the sheep model, which may more accurately represent the human situation because brain maturation is more precocial, overfeeding of ewes during pregnancy seems to alter anorexigenic mechanisms that work through the appetite-inhibiting cocaine and amphetamineregulated transcript [44–46].

Subcutaneous leptin administration in the early neonatal period stimulates the outgrowth of neurons in the developing neonatal rat hypothalamus from the arcuate nucleus to innervate the paraventricular nucleus in a manner that enhances development of neuropeptide Y and agouti-related protein connections to the paraventricular nucleus in preference to from appetite inhibitory αMSH projections [47,48]. Several studies have been conducted to elucidate the timing and detailed development of the effects of leptin on the rodent hypothalamic architecture. Leptin injected subcutaneously to neonatal rats on days 3 to 13 of neonatal life reversed the ability of prenatal undernutrition to produce offspring hyperphagia and obesity [49]. In contrast, in other studies, offspring obesity has been associated with a premature leptin surge in mice. The normal rise in leptin in the neonatal period occurs approximately 16 days postnatal life [50]. Maternal undernutrition that results in offspring obesity is associated with an earlier offspring neonatal leptin surge—approximately 8 to 10 days. Leptin administration to mice in early postnatal life produces offspring obesity [50]. It therefore seems that several different alterations of the precise timing of exposure of the central appetite regulating systems to leptin can alter the set point of activity of both the orexigenic and anorexigenic systems. Further studies need to be conducted to determine the interplay and precise timing of the developmental programming mechanisms, including potential roles for hypercorstisolaemia and hyperinsulinaemia, which have also been implicated [51].

Although no studies have been conducted on the effects of maternal obesity and offspring physical activity, one study on the effects of maternal nutrient restriction on physical activity of offspring clearly shows that the level of an individual's physical activity can be programmed by maternal nutrition. A severe nutrient restriction paradigm in the rat, in which the maternal diet is reduced by 90% compared with controls throughout pregnancy followed by a normal diet during lactation, produced offspring that were obese and undertook much less wheel running than offspring of control mothers [52,53]. When the offspring of the undernourished mothers were fed a high-fat diet, they indulged in even less physical activity. There is evidence that the composition of lipids in the maternal diet may also be important. Offspring of rats fed a lard-rich diet containing mostly saturated fats showed decreased physical activity [54]. In contrast, when pregnant mice are fed a diet rich in polyunsaturated fat, offspring show increased swim test activity [55].

## Altered development of adipose tissue

Raised maternal plasma glucose concentrations occur in situations of maternal adiposity and gestational diabetes. Infusion of glucose into the ovine fetus results in increased fetal fat mass [56]. An increased fat mass is also present in weanling rats of mothers fed a highly palatable diet in pregnancy and lactation [57] and in adult offspring of rats fed a fat-rich diet [58–60]. There is increasing evidence that altered maternal nutritional states can program important cell, gene, and enzyme functions that play key roles in adipogenesis and adipocyte function. Increased expression of 11βHSD-1, a key enzyme that controls the local availability of cortisol, has been demonstrated in the adipose tissue of lambs that were nutrient-restricted before birth [61]. Cortisol plays a key role in the development of fetal adipose tissue. Another family of regulators of adipose tissue development is the peroxisome proliferator-activated receptors (PPAR). These are transcription factor members of the nuclear receptor superfamily. PPARα and γ have been shown to be altered in adipose tissue and liver of offspring of rats fed a low-protein diet [62]. Indeed adipose tissue gene expression profiling by microarray has revealed several molecular pathways that may contribute to adiposity in offspring of protein-restricted dams [63]. In the fetal liver, the expression of PPARα has been shown to depend on folic acid availability and thus methylation status [64]. Recently, Muhlhausler and colleagues [44] have shown an increase in expression of PPARγ, lipoprotein lipase, adiponectin, and leptin mRNA expression in the fetal prerenal fat of lambs whose dams were fed a diet 55% above energy maintenance requirements; the data suggests a precocial increase in pathways, which could contribute to obesity in later life.

## Altered insulin secretion and resistance

It has been known for many years that maternal nutrient status and particularly maternal hyperglycemia alters the development of the fetal pancreas. Thus increased glucose transport from mother to fetus results in exposure of the developing fetal pancreas to higher than normal glucose levels with a resultant acceleration of pancreatic development. The authors' data show an increase in fetal insulin levels in sheep fetuses of mothers eating 150% of nutrient requirement consumed by controls for the first half of pregnancy [65]. This accelerated maturation appears to predispose the pancreas of the offspring to fail when exposed to challenges in later life. The authors and others have also shown that adult offspring of lard-fed dams demonstrate structural and functional evidence for pancreatic beta cell dysfunction [60,66].

The exact nature of fatty acid exposure to which a developing fetus is exposed will depend on both the level of maternal adiposity and the fat composition of her diet. Offspring of dams fed a diet rich in saturated fats develop insulin resistance in adulthood [58,60,66], whereas feeding mothers polyunsaturated fats does not produce insulin resistance in offspring [67]. The importance of the ratio of different fatty acids, especially the polyunsaturated fatty acids, has been elegantly demonstrated in one study in which offspring of mothers fed a high n-6:n-3 ratio diet in soybean oil had raised fasting insulin and increased fat deposition in adult life [68]. These effects of maternal obesity and diet may program female offspring so that they themselves demonstrate gestational diabetes during their own pregnancy and pass the predisposition across generations from daughter to granddaughter [69–72].

Weanling rats born to mothers fed on a highly palatable obesogenic cafeteria diet during pregnancy and lactation have smaller skeletal muscles with fewer muscle fibers compared with offspring of rats fed the normal diet. Increased intramuscular lipid content and adipocyte hypertrophy were also present [57]. Because insulin sensitivity is greatly dependent on an adequate skeletal muscle mass, and muscle lipid content is directly related to insulin resistance [73], these consequences of overnutrition during development could increase the offspring's predisposition to insulin resistance in later life.

## Altered cardiovascular function

Altered cardiovascular function resulting from deficient maternal diets was amongst the first convincing demonstrations of developmental programming in animal models [53,74–79]. Most of the early studies investigated the effects of maternal low-protein diets [80]. However, raised blood pressure was observed in offspring of rats fed a coconut oil–rich diet and in the offspring of rat dams fed a diet rich in soybean oil [68]. Endothelial dysfunction has been reported in offspring of dams subjected to dietary restriction or protein deprivation [74,81–83]. In one of the authors' studies, maternal overnutrition resulted in hypertension only in female offspring, whereas both males and females exhibit blunted endothelium-dependent relaxation [54].

## Implications for the future

The evidence presented on the mechanisms by which maternal obesity and gestational diabetes predispose offspring to subsequent chronic disease indicates the extreme importance of these conditions in pregnancy. It is imperative that further information is obtained to provide evidence-based strategies to decrease the incidence of obesity in women of child-bearing years, recommend optimal diets suited to the phenotype of each individual pregnant woman, and improve management during pregnancy.

## References

[1] ACOG Committee opinion number 315. Obesity in pregnancy. Obstet Gynecol 2005;106: 671–5.
[2] Hedley AA, Ogden CL, Johnson CL, et al. Prevalence of overweight and obesity among US children, adolescents, and adults, 1999–2002. JAMA 2004;291:2847–50.
[3] Ogden CL, Carroll MD, Curtin LR, et al. Prevalence of overweight and obesity in the United States, 1999–2004. JAMA 2006;295:1549–55.
[4] Villamor E, Cnattingiusl S. Interpregnancy weight change and risk of adverse pregnancy outcomes: a population-based study. Lancet 2006;368:1164–70.
[5] Armitage JA, Khan IY, Taylor PD, et al. Developmental programming of the metabolic syndrome by maternal nutritional imbalance: how strong is the evidence from experimental models in mammals? J Physiol 2004;561:355–77.
[6] Armitage JA, Taylor PD, Poston L. Experimental models of developmental programming: consequences of exposure to an energy rich diet during development. J Physiol 2005;565: 3–8.
[7] Armitage JA, Ishibashi A, Balachandran AA, et al. Programmed aortic dysfunction and reduced Na+, K+ATPase activity present in first generation offspring of lard-fed rats does not persist to the second generation. Exp Physiol 2007;92(3):583–9.
[8] Gluckman PD, Hanson MA, Beedle AS. Non-genomic transgenerational inheritance of disease risk. Bioessays 2007;29:145–54.
[9] McMillen IC, Robinson JS. Developmental origins of the metabolic syndrome: prediction, plasticity, and programming. Physiol Rev 2005;85:571–633.
[10] Nathanielsz PW. Animal models that elucidate basic principles of the developmental origins of adult diseases. Ilar News 2006;47(1):73–82.
[11] Gluckman PD, Hanson MA. The developmental origins of the metabolic syndrome. Trends Endocrinol Metab 2004;15:183–7.
[12] Barker DJ, Osmond C. Infant mortality: childhood nutrition and ischaemic heart disease in England and Wales. Lancet 1986;1:1077–81.
[13] Barker DJP. Mothers, babies and health in later life. 2nd edition. Edinburgh (Scotland): Churchill Livingstone; 1998.
[14] Newsome CA, Shiell AW, Fall CHD, et al. Is birth weight related to later glucose and insulin metabolism?—a systematic review. Diabet Med 2003;20:339–48.
[15] Barker DJP, Osmond C, Forsen TJ, et al. Trajectories of growth among children who have coronary events as adults. N Engl J Med 2005;353:1802–9.
[16] Bhargava SK, Sachdev HS, Fall CHD, et al. Relation of serial changes in childhood body-mass index to impaired glucose tolerance in young adulthood. N Engl J Med 2004;350: 865–75.
[17] Eriksson JG, Forsen T, Tuomilehto J, et al. Early adiposity rebound in childhood and risk of type 2 diabetes in adult life. Diabetologia 2003;46:190–4.
[18] Singhal A, Lucas A. Early origins of cardiovascular disease: is there a unifying hypothesis? Lancet 2004;363:1642–5.
[19] Catalano PM, Ehrenberg HM. The short- and long-term implications of maternal obesity on the mother and her offspring. BJOG 2006;113:1126–33.
[20] Jennifer S Huang, Tiffany AL, Michael CL. Prenatal programming of childhood overweight and obesity. Matern Child Health J 2006;Sept. 28 [epub ahead of print].
[21] Catalano PM, Thomas A, Huston-Presley L, et al. Increased fetal adiposity: a very sensitive marker of abnormal in utero development. Am J Obstet Gynecol 2003;189:1698–704.

[22] Catalano PM. Obesity and pregnancy—the propagation of a viscous cycle? J Clin Endocrinol Metab 2003;88:3505–6.

[23] Oken E, Gillman MW. Fetal origins of obesity. Obes Res 2003;11:496–506.

[24] Salsberry PJ, Reagan PB. Dynamics of early childhood overweight. Pediatrics 2005;116: 1329–38.

[25] Harder T, Rodekamp E, Schellong K, et al. Birth weight and subsequent risk of type 2 diabetes: a meta-analysis. Am J Epidemiol 2007;165(8):849–57.

[26] Curhan GC, Chertow GM, Willett WC, et al. Birth weight and adult hypertension and obesity in women. Circulation 1996;94:1310–5.

[27] Rogers I. Birth weight and obesity and fat distribution in later life. Clinical and Molecular Birth Defects Res A Clin Mol Teratol 2005;73(7):485–6.

[28] Schaefer-Graf UM, Pawliczak J, Passow D, et al. Birth weight and parental BMI predict overweight in children from mothers with gestational diabetes. Diabetes Care 2005;28: 1745–50.

[29] Dorner G. Perinatal hyperinsulinism as possible predisposing factor for diabetes mellitus, obesity and enhanced cardiovascular risk in later life. Horm Metab Res 1994;26:213–21.

[30] Dabelea D. Intrauterine diabetic environment confers risks for type 2 diabetes mellitus and obesity in the offspring, in addition to genetic susceptibility. J Pediatr Endocrinol Metab 2001;14:1085–91.

[31] Dabelea D, Hanson RL, Lindsay RS, et al. Intrauterine exposure to diabetes conveys risks for type 2 diabetes and obesity: a study of discordant sibships. Diabetes 2000;49:2208–11.

[32] Boney CM, Verma A, Tucker R, et al. Metabolic syndrome in childhood: association with birth weight, maternal obesity, and gestational diabetes mellitus. Pediatrics 2005;115: e290–6.

[33] Sacks DA, Liu AI, Wolde-Tsadik G, et al. What proportion of birth weight is attributable to maternal glucose among infants of diabetic women? Am J Obstet Gynecol 2006;194: 501–7.

[34] Singhal A, Wells J, Cole TJ, et al. Programming of lean body mass: a link between birth weight, obesity, and cardiovascular disease? Am J Clin Nutr 2003;77:726–30.

[35] Sewell MF, Huston-Presley L, Super DM, et al. Increased neonatal fat mass, not lean body mass, is associated with maternal obesity. Am J Obstet Gynecol 2006;195:1100–3.

[36] Lewis DS. Preweaning food intake influences the adiposity of young adult baboons. J Clin Invest 1986;78:899–905.

[37] Plagemann A. Perinatal programming and functional teratogenesis: impact on body weight regulation and obesity. Physiol Behav 2005;86:661–8.

[38] Grove KL, Smith MS. Ontogeny of the hypothalamic neuropeptide Y system. Physiol Behav 2003;79:47–63.

[39] Grayson BE, Allen SE, Billes SK, et al. Prenatal development of hypothalamic neuropeptide systems in the nonhuman primate. Neuroscience 2006;143:975–86.

[40] Plagemann A. Elevation of hypothalamic neuropeptide Y-neurons in adult offspring of diabetic mother rats. Neuroreport 1999;10:3211–6.

[41] Schmidt I, Fritz A, Scholch C, et al. The effect of leptin treatment on the development of obesity in overfed suckling Wistar rats. Int J Obes 2001;25:1168–74.

[42] Kozak R, Burlet A, Burlet C, et al. Dietary composition during fetal and neonatal life affects neuropeptide Y functioning in adult offspring. Brain Res Dev Brain Res 2000;125:75–82.

[43] Beck B, Kozak R, Moar KM, et al. Hypothalamic orexigenic peptides are overexpressed in young Long-Evans rats after early life exposure to fat-rich diets. Biochem Biophys Res Commun 2006;342:452–8.

[44] Muhlhausler BS. Programming of the appetite-regulating neural network: a link between maternal overnutrition and the programming of obesity? J Neuroendocrinol 2007;19: 67–72.

[45] Muhlhausler BS, Adam CL, Marrocco EM, et al. Impact of glucose infusion on the structural and functional characteristics of adipose tissue and on hypothalamic gene expression

for appetite regulatory neuropeptides in the sheep fetus during late gestation. J Physiol 2005; 565:185–95.

[46] Muhlhausler BS, Findlay PA, Duffield JA, et al. Increased maternal nutrition alters development of the appetite-regulating network in the brain. FASEB J 2006;20(8):1257–9.

[47] Bouret SG, Draper SJ, Simerly RB. Trophic action of leptin on hypothalamic neurons that regulate feeding. Science 2004;304:108–10.

[48] Horvath TL, Bruning JC. Developmental programming of the hypothalamus: a matter of fat. Nat Med 2006;12:52–3.

[49] Vickers MH, Gluckman PD, Coveny AH, et al. Neonatal leptin treatment reverses developmental programming. Endocrinology 2005;146:4211–6.

[50] Yura S, Itoh H, Sagawa N, et al. Role of premature leptin surge in obesity resulting from intrauterine undernutrition. Cell Metab 2005;1:371–8.

[51] Plagemann A. Perinatal nutrition and hormone-dependent programming of food intake. Horm Res 2006;65(Suppl 3):83–9.

[52] Vickers MH, Breier BH, McCarthy D, et al. Sedentary behavior during postnatal life is determined by the prenatal environment and exacerbated by postnatal hypercaloric nutrition. Am J Physiol Regul Integr Comp Physiol 2003;285:R271–3.

[53] Vickers MH, Breier BH, Cutfield WS, et al. Fetal origins of hyperphagia, obesity, and hypertension and postnatal amplification by hypercaloric nutrition. Am J Physiol Endocrinol Metab 2000;279:E83–7.

[54] Khan IY, Taylor PD, Dekou V, et al. Gender-linked hypertension in offspring of lard-fed pregnant rats. Hypertension 2003;41:168–75.

[55] Raygada M, Cho E, Hilakivi-Clarke L. High maternal intake of polyunsaturated fatty acids during pregnancy in mice alters offsprings' aggressive behavior, immobility in the swim test, locomotor activity and brain protein kinase C activity. J Nutr 1998;128: 2505–11.

[56] Stevens D, Alexander G, Bell AW. Effect of prolonged glucose infusion into fetal sheep on body growth, fat deposition and gestation length. J Dev Physiol 1990;13:277–81.

[57] Bayol SA, Simbi BH, Stickland NC. A maternal cafeteria diet during gestation and lactation promotes adiposity and impairs skeletal muscle development and metabolism in rat offspring at weaning. J Physiol 2005;567:951–61.

[58] Buckley AJ, Keseru B, Briody J, et al. Altered body composition and metabolism in the male offspring of high fat-fed rats. Metabolism 2005;54:500–7.

[59] Khan IY, Dekou V, Douglas G, et al. A high-fat diet during rat pregnancy or suckling induces cardiovascular dysfunction in adult offspring. Am J Physiol Regul Integr Comp Physiol 2005;288:R127–33.

[60] Srinivasan M, Katewa SD, Palaniyappan A, et al. Maternal high-fat diet consumption results in fetal malprogramming predisposing to the onset of metabolic syndrome-like phenotype in adulthood. Am J Physiol Endocrinol Metab 2006;291:E792–9.

[61] Whorwood CB, Firth KM, Budge H, et al. Maternal undernutrition during early to midgestation programs tissue-specific alterations in the expression of the glucocorticoid receptor, 11β-hydroxysteroid dehydrogenase isoforms, and type-1 angiotensin II receptor in neonatal sheep. Endocrinology 2001;142(2001):2854–64.

[62] Desai M, Gayle D, Babu J, et al. Programmed obesity in intrauterine growth-restricted newborns: modulation by newborn nutrition. Am J Physiol Regul Integr Comp Physiol 2005;288:R91–6.

[63] Guan H, Arany E, van Beek JP, et al. Adipose tissue gene expression profiling reveals distinct molecular pathways that define visceral adiposity in offspring of maternal protein-restricted rats. Am J Physiol Endocrinol Metab 2005;288:E663–73.

[64] Lillycrop KA, Phillips ES, Jackson AA, et al. Dietary protein restriction of pregnant rats induces and folic acid supplementation prevents epigenetic modification of hepatic gene expression in the offspring. J Nutr 2005;135:1382–6.

[65] Ford SP, Miller MM, Hess B, et al. Impact of maternal obesity on growth and pancreatic function in the fetal sheep [abstract]. J Soc Gynecol Investig Reprod Sciences 2007;14(1): 238A.

[66] Taylor PD, McConnell J, Khan IY, et al. Impaired glucose homeostasis and mitochondrial abnormalities in offspring of rats fed a fat-rich diet in pregnancy. Am J Physiol Regul Integr Comp Physiol 2005;288:R134–9.

[67] Siemelink M, Verhoef A, Dormans JA, et al. Dietary fatty acid composition during pregnancy and lactation in the rat programs growth and glucose metabolism in the offspring. Diabetologia 2002;45:1397–403.

[68] Korotkova M, Gabrielsson BG, Holmang A, et al. Gender-related long-term effects in adult rats by perinatal dietary ratio of n-6/n-3 fatty acids. Am J Physiol Regul Integr Comp Physiol 2005;288:R575–9.

[69] Zambrano E, Bautista CJ, Deas M, et al. A low maternal protein diet during pregnancy and lactation has sex- and window of exposure-specific effects on offspring growth and food intake, glucose metabolism and serum leptin in the rat. J Physiol 2006;571:221–30.

[70] Zambrano E, Rodriguez-Gonzalez GL, Guzman C, et al. A maternal low protein diet during pregnancy and lactation in the rat impairs male reproductive development. J Physiol 2005; 563:275–84.

[71] Zambrano E, Nathanielsz PW, McDonald TJ. Prenatal and postnatal ovine adrenal cell responses to prostaglandin E2. Journal of the Society for Gynecological Investigations 2001;8:149–57.

[72] Zambrano E, Martinez-Samayoa PM, Bautista CJ, et al. Sex differences in transgenerational alterations of growth and metabolism in progeny (F2) of female offspring (F1) of rats fed a low protein diet during pregnancy and lactation. J Physiol 2005;566:225–36.

[73] Savage DB, Petersen KF, Shulman GI. Mechanisms of insulin resistance in humans and possible links with inflammation. Hypertension 2005;45:828–33.

[74] Brawley L, Itoh S, Torrens C, et al. Dietary protein restriction in pregnancy induces hypertension and vascular defects in rat male offspring. Pediatr Res 2003;54:83–90.

[75] Franco MC, Dantas AP, Akaminnme EH, et al. Enhanced oxidative stress as a potential mechanism underlying the programming of hypertension in utero. J Cardiovascular Pharmcol 2002;40:501–9.

[76] Langley S, Jackson AA. Increased systolic blood pressure in adult rats induced by fetal exposure to maternal low protein diets. Clin Sci 1994;86:217–22.

[77] Ozaki T, Nishina H, Hanson MA, et al. Dietary restriction in pregnant rats causes gender-related hypertension and vascular dysfunction in offspring. J Physiol 2001;530:141–52.

[78] Tonkiss J, Trzcinska M, Galler JR, et al. Prenatal malnutrition-induced changes in blood pressure: dissociation of stress and nonstress responses using radiotelemetry. Hypertension 1998;32:108–14.

[79] Woods LL, Ingelfinger JR, Nyengaard JR, et al. Maternal protein restriction suppresses the newborn renin-angiotensin system and programs adult hypertension in rats. Pediatr Res 2001;49:460–7.

[80] Langley-Evans SC, Clamp AG, Grimble RF, et al. Influence of dietary fats upon systolic blood pressure in the rat. Int J Food Sci and Nutr 1996;47:417–25.

[81] Holemans K. Maternal food restriction in the second half of pregnancy affects vascular function but not blood pressure of rat female offspring. Br J Nutr 1999;81:73–9.

[82] Lamireau D, Nuyt AM, Hou X, et al. Altered vascular function in fetal programming of hypertension. Stroke 2002;33:2992–8.

[83] Torrens C, Brawley L, Barker AC, et al. Maternal protein restriction in the rat impairs resistance artery but not conduit artery function in pregnant offspring. J Physiol 2003;547: 77–84.

ELSEVIER
SAUNDERS

Obstet Gynecol Clin N Am
34 (2007) 213–224

OBSTETRICS AND
GYNECOLOGY
CLINICS
OF NORTH AMERICA

# Inflammatory Mediators
# in Gestational Diabetes Mellitus

## Alvie C. Richardson, MD,
## Marshall W. Carpenter, MD*

*Division of Maternal Fetal Medicine, Department of Obstetrics and Gynecology,*
*Women and Infants' Hospital of Rhode Island/Brown University School of Medicine,*
*3rd Floor, Providence, RI 02905, USA*

Pregnancy is characterized by an increase in insulin resistance. Hyperglycemia is avoided secondary to a compensatory increase in insulin production by the pancreatic beta-cell. However, when the pancreatic beta-cell
fails to compensate sufficiently, glucose metabolism is altered and gestational diabetes mellitus (GDM) develops. The primary etiology of the rise
in insulin resistance during normal pregnancy has long been thought to be
endocrine in nature and associated with gestational hormones. However, recent evidence has demonstrated that tumor necrosis factor-alpha (TNF-α),
an inflammatory cytokine, may be a better predictor of insulin resistance in
pregnancy than gestational hormones [1]. This finding challenges the perspective that gestational hormones are the sole contributor to insulin resistance in pregnancy and suggests a possible relationship with inflammatory
mediators. Although the association between inflammation and GDM is
a new finding, the connection between inflammation and insulin resistance
is well known and is supported by epidemiologic as well as clinical data.
This article reviews the current evidence supporting the link between inflammation and GDM.

## Glucose metabolism in normal pregnancy

Normal pregnancy is marked by significant changes in maternal fuel
homeostasis. Early pregnancy is associated with a decrease in fasting
plasma glucose concentrations [2] and a slight decrease in basal endogenous

---

* Corresponding author.
*E-mail address:* mcarpent@wihri.org (M.W. Carpenter).

0889-8545/07/$ - see front matter © 2007 Elsevier Inc. All rights reserved.
doi:10.1016/j.ogc.2007.04.001

glucose production [3]. However, by the end of the first trimester, insulin sensitivity starts to fall, and by the third trimester, insulin-stimulated glucose disposal has been shown to decline by approximately 50% in lean [4] and by 40% in obese women [5]. This has been associated with accelerated ketosis in the fasting state and an increase in maternal fasting glucose and free fatty acids.

The cause of the first-trimester insulin sensitivity rise is unknown. The subsequent fall of insulin sensitivity (rise in resistance) is likely the result of several stimuli. A rise in plasma concentrations of several hormones, such as chorionic somatomamotropin (placental lactogen), progesterone, prolactin, and cortisol, have been observed to correlate with the development of midpregnancy insulin resistance and their fall with postpartum changes. However, the correlation of insulin resistance with endocrine change may reflect other intermediate mechanisms. Serum concentration of TNF-α, an inflammatory cytokine produced by cells of the immune system, has also been linked with insulin resistance in pregnancy. Kirwan and colleagues [1] reported that circulating concentrations of TNF-α were inversely proportional to insulin sensitivity when measured by euglycemic-hyperinsulinemic clamp studies. Furthermore, when compared with other pregnancy-related hormones (leptin, cortisol, placental lactogen, human chorionic gonadotropin, estradiol, progesterone, and prolactin), the change in plasma TNF-α concentration from the pregravid state to late pregnancy was the best predictor of insulin sensitivity [1].

The observed increase in insulin resistance that characterizes midpregnancy is met with a compensatory increase in fasting and postmeal plasma insulin concentrations due to increased insulin production by the pancreatic beta-cell. The pancreatic beta-cell's ability to produce enough insulin in the face of increasing insulin resistance is a necessary requirement to maintain euglycemia in normal pregnancy.

## Pathophysiology of gestational diabetes mellitus

GDM is defined as carbohydrate intolerance first recognized during pregnancy [6]. GDM is a unique physiologic state that is distinguishable from the normal metabolic changes induced by pregnancy. Compared to normal pregnancy, GDM is characterized by increased insulin resistance. Evidence to support greater insulin resistance in GDM versus nondiabetic pregnancy is provided by Xiang and colleagues [7], who by using the hyperinsulinemic-euglycemic clamp technique demonstrated reduced suppression of basal glucose production and reduced insulin-mediated glucose clearance among women who have GDM in response to similar elevations of plasma insulin. Similarly, Catalano and colleagues [8] used the same method to demonstrate, among obese gravidas, that those who developed GDM had higher insulin resistance throughout gestation. It has been suggested that the greater magnitude of insulin resistance in GDM is likely due to the additive nature of chronic underlying insulin resistance superimposed upon that due to normal pregnancy [9]. Because the incidence of GDM has a strong association with maternal obesity [10], the pathogenesis of GDM is likely that of chronic insulin resistance due to increased fat mass. Additionally, genetically determined insulin signaling dysfunction may also contribute to insulin resistance and may lead, in some cases, to GDM. Friedman and colleagues [11] described that those who have GDM have a distinct decrease in the ability of the insulin receptor-beta to undergo tyrosine phosphorylation compared to those with non-diabetic pregnancy. This defect was associated with lower glucose transport activity in comparison to nondiabetic gravidas [11].

Pancreatic beta-cell dysfunction is the other key feature observed in those who have GDM. Homko and colleagues [12] determined that beta-cell function is decreased by 41% during pregnancy and 50% after pregnancy among those who have GDM compared with controls. Beta-cell dysfunction can occur secondary to autoimmunity directed against the pancreatic beta-cell, monogenic origins such as maturity-onset diabetes of the young or in the setting of chronic insulin resistance. Due to its common association with obesity, it is likely that most of those who have GDM have beta-cell dysfunction arising on a background of chronic insulin resistance secondary to obesity.

Although beta-cell dysfunction is clearly occurring on a background of chronic insulin resistance, the actual mechanism by which beta-cell failure develops is unclear. The pancreatic-beta cell initially responds to insulin resistance by expanding beta-cell mass to produce enough insulin to meet physiologic demand. Butler and colleagues [13], using autopsy specimens, observed increased beta-cell mass among obese but nondiabetic subjects. In contrast, those who had a combination of obesity and type 2 diabetes mellitus (T2DM) demonstrated decreased beta-cell mass. The authors speculated that their findings reflected increased beta-cell apoptosis. If the cause of decreased beta-cell mass was related to chronic increased beta-cell "demand," then reduction of insulin resistance may delay the development of clinically significant hyperglycemia. This hypothesis has been supported by Buchanan and colleagues [14], who conducted a placebo controlled randomized trial of troglitazone among nonpregnant women who had a recent history of GDM. Troglitazone is a drug known to reduce insulin resistance and possess anti-inflammatory properties. During a median follow-up of 30 months, the average annual diabetes incidence rates were 12.1% versus 5.4% in women assigned to placebo and troglitazone, respectively. The reduction in diabetes was attributed to preservation of pancreatic beta-cell function and appeared to be mediated by a reduction in the secretory demands placed upon the beta-cells by chronic insulin resistance. These findings and conclusions were further supported by a proglitazone trial by the same investigators [15].

## The immune system and inflammatory mediators

The immune system defends its host against both external threats, such as bacterial infection, viral infection; physical injury, and internal threats such as malignant transformation. The immune system has historically been divided into two parts: the innate and adaptive. They are separated purely for descriptive purposes and are not mutually exclusive of one another. From an evolutionary standpoint, the innate immune system predates the adaptive immune system. The innate immune system is considered to be the "first-line" of defense against microbes or tissue damage. The adaptive immune system is activated by the innate immune system and responds to antigens to which the organism has already been exposed, thereby providing the ability to mount a more effective response.

Innate immune function involves direct recognition of pathogens by relying upon a limited number of germline-encoded pattern recognition receptors, better known as Toll-receptors, which are possessed by all innate immune cells. These receptors evolved to recognize highly conserved microbial polysacchride and polynucleotide patterns and are collectively described as pathogen-associated molecular patterns. Pathogen-associated molecular patterns are not possessed by the host. Recognition of these molecular structures allows the immune system to distinguish nonself from self.

The cells of the innate immune system are present in all tissues, and they include mast cells, phagocytes (macrophages, dendritic cells, polymorphonuclear leukocytes), basophils, eosinophils, natural killer cells, and gamma delta T-cells. Once bound by pathogen-associated molecular patterns, the pattern recognition receptors trigger the innate immune cell to directly destroy the pathogen; process an antigen for presentation; and/or activate a signaling pathway that induces antimicrobial genes, which results in the production and release of inflammatory mediators known as cytokines. Cytokines are proteins and are functionally similar to classical endocrine hormones. Cytokines mediate signaling between cells and are produced by cells of the immune system as well as a few other cell types such as adipocytes and endothelial cells. Cytokines can act locally but also circulate and exert their effects systemically. Once the cytokine is bound to a specific immune cell-surface receptor, intracellular signaling events initiate, perpetuate, and/or down-regulate immunologic responses. Cytokines can, however, bind non-immunologic cells resulting in several different effects, one of which is cellular response to insulin.

### Cytokines and insulin resistance

Cytokines exert their effect upon insulin resistance by interfering with the insulin receptor–signaling cascade. The insulin receptor is a protein tyrosine kinase that upon binding insulin, results in the phosphorylation of intracellular substrates. Upon phosphorylation, these substrates interact and activate other molecules that modulate intracellular metabolism. Cytokines can directly interfere with the intracellular signaling cascade of the insulin receptor. For example, TNF-α, an inflammatory cytokine, can induce insulin resistance by decreasing serine phosphorylation of the insulin receptor kinase [16]. TNF-α has also been shown to promote serine phosphorylation of insulin receptor substrate-1, which in turn effectively blocks insulin receptor substrate-1 from binding to the insulin receptor [17]. Interleukin-6, another inflammatory cytokine, also induces insulin resistance by inhibiting glucose transporter-4 synthesis as well as up-regulating suppressor of cytokine -3, which inhibits tyrosine phosphorylation of insulin receptor substrate-1 and -2 [18,19].

### Obesity, inflammation, and insulin resistance

Obesity is rapidly rising to epidemic proportions worldwide including the United States. According to the most recent National Health Examination Survey in 2003 to 2004, the prevalence of obesity in reproductive aged women 20 to 39 years old in the United States, defined as a body mass index (BMI) $\geq$ 30 kg/m2, was 28.9% [20]. In addition to its other related morbidities, obesity observed is associated with an increased risk for GDM [21–23]. Baeten and colleagues [24] identified an association between obesity (BMI $\geq$ 30) and GDM with an odds ratio of 5.2 (4.3, 6.2) among a geographic sample of 96,801 nulliparous women. Furthermore, fetal exposure to maternal obesity increases the risk of childhood metabolic syndrome (obesity, hypertension, glucose intolerance, and dyslipidemia) approximately twofold [25]. This would suggest that maternal adiposity may affect fetal metabolic programming.

Adipose tissue is no longer considered a passive tissue solely used for lipid storage. Rather, it is a diverse tissue that also actively participates in endocrine and immune functions. The remarkable ability of adipose tissue to function as an endocrine organ and as an immune organ reflects the character of its precursor cell, the preadipocyte. The preadipocyte has the ability to differentiate and mature into an adipocyte or a macrophage [26]. This differentiation is likely secondary to the metabolic or immunologic demands placed upon the cell. The adipocyte mediates its effects by way of proteins called adipokines that influence not only adipocyte-related autocrine and paracrine function, but also modulate local and systemic immune cell functions and systemic metabolic pathways. Altered adipokine production, particularly those possessing inflammatory properties, has been associated with obesity-associated insulin resistance.

TNF-α, an inflammatory cytokine, is an adipokine that induces inflammation by inhibiting production of adiponectin, an anti-inflammatory adipokine [27]; recruits other inflammatory cells of the innate immune system; and stimulates release of free fatty acids [28]. TNF-α's association with obesity and insulin resistance was first recognized by Hotamisligil and colleagues [29] in 1993. They were able to demonstrate higher TNF-α concentrations in plasma and adipose tissue in obese versus lean mice. Furthermore, when the neutralized TNF-α, they were able to see a reduction of insulin resistance. In humans, serum concentrations of TNF-α have been found to be elevated in obese individuals, and subsequent weight loss leads to decreased serum concentrations [30]. These trends are also observed in human adipose tissue. Hotamisligil and colleagues [31] demonstrated greater expression of TNF-α messenger RNA in adipose tissue of obese individuals in comparison to nonobese individuals, and weight reduction resulted in a decrease expression of TNF-α messenger RNA and a subsequent improvement in insulin sensitivity.

Interleukin-6, another inflammatory cytokine, is produced by the adipocyte and is key stimulator of acute phase proteins (C-reactive protein, amyloid A, complement, and so forth) production by the human hepatocyte [32]. In humans, elevated plasma concentrations of interleukin-6 are associated with obesity [33,34] and insulin resistance, even when controlling for BMI [33]. Similar to TNF-α, weight loss is associated with a reduction in interleukin-6 concentration in serum [33,34]. Interleukin-6, when administered to healthy individuals, increases blood glucose in a dose-dependent manner [35]. The mechanism by which this occurs is unknown.

Adiponectin is an anti-inflammatory adipokine. Adiponectin mediates its anti-inflammatory effects by inhibiting macrophage phagocytic capabilities, TNF-α induced expression of adhesion molecules [36], as well as TNF-α production from macrophages [37]. Adiponectin mRNA is reduced in adipose tissue in obese humans [38]. Plasma concentrations of adiponectin are also lower in obese individuals [39] and rise with weight loss [40]. In cross-sectional studies of humans, plasma adiponectin levels are negatively correlated with insulin resistance [39]. Further, adiponectin administration in rodent models of obesity and T2DM reverses insulin resistance [41]. The mechanism of this effect has not been identified.

## Pregnancy and the immune system

Normal pregnancy is accompanied by alterations within the maternal innate and adaptive immune system. The maternal innate immune system seems to be stimulated in pregnancy, whereas the adaptive immune system is believed to be relatively suppressed [42]. Systemically this is manifest as an increase in the number of circulating innate immune cells, such as monocytes and granulocytes, which have been shown to possess activated phenotypes comparable to those observed in sepsis [43]. Plasma concentrations of inflammatory cytokine TNF-α [1], acute-phase proteins, C-reactive protein [44], fibrinogen, and complement [45] are increased in pregnancy. The innate immune system also seems to be up-regulated locally, at the level of the utero-placental interface, in which there are increased numbers of uterine natural killer cells, macrophages, and gamma delta T cells [46]. The maternal adaptive immune system, on the other hand, seems to be suppressed, particularly at the utero-placental interface [47], as evidenced by diminished B and T cells. It has been opined that these changes allow for successful immuno-tolerance of paternally derived antigens of the fetal allograft.

## Gestational diabetes mellitus and inflammation

Evidence of inflammatory dysregulation can be observed as early as the first trimester among gravidas who later develop GDM. Wolf and colleagues [48], in a prospective cohort of 2753 nulliparous euglycemic women, identified increased leukocyte count ($10.5 \pm 2.2$ versus $9.2 \pm 2.2 \times 10^3$ cells/mL; $P < .01$) in early pregnancy among those who had subsequent GDM independent of BMI. These findings are consistent with other studies outside of pregnancy that have observed leukocyte count to be a predictor in the development of T2DM [49,50].

Several cytokines have been linked to insulin resistance observed in those who had GDM. Kirwan and colleagues [1] noted significantly higher third-trimester serum TNF-$\alpha$ concentration among obese individuals who had GDM when compared with lean controls ($2.84 \pm 0.17$ versus $2.13 \pm 0.17$ pg/mL; $P < .02$). Moreover, the increase of TNF-$\alpha$ concentration from pregravid to the third trimester was the best predictor of insulin resistance in pregnancy when compared with leptin, cortisol, and other pregnancy-derived hormones (placental lactogen, human chorionic gonadotropin, estradiol, progesterone, and prolactin) independent of fat mass [1]. Similarly, Ategbo and colleagues [51] demonstrated serum concentrations of TNF-$\alpha$ and interleukin-6, to be elevated at time of delivery in those who had GDM, though no attempt was made to control for fat mass.

A decreased anti-inflammatory response has also been identified among those who have GDM. Specifically, first-trimester plasma concentrations of adiponectin, an anti-inflammatory adipokine, have been found to be statistically lower in women who develop GDM, independent of risk factors for GDM [52]. Serum concentrations of interleukin-10, an anti-inflammatory cytokine, in the third trimester have been found to be lower in those who have GDM independent of obesity [53]. This finding is consistent with previous studies describing an association between low plasma interleukin-10 levels and the metabolic syndrome [54]. Furthermore, the ability of immune cells to produce interleukin-10 in response to an inflammatory stimulus is blunted in those who have GDM when compared with matched controls [53]. This finding is also consistent with previous studies linking low interleukin-10 production capability with T2DM in the elderly population [55]. These findings would suggest that the cytokine profile in those who have GDM is best characterized as an imbalance between inflammatory and anti-inflammatory mediators.

Placentas among those who have GDM also display the presence of an inflammatory state. Radaelli and colleagues [56] examined the profile of gene expression in human placentas obtained from normal and GDM pregnancies and found that genes regulating inflammatory responses were altered in those who had GDM. Specifically, up-regulation of genes for interleukins, leptin, and TNF-α receptors and their downstream molecular adaptors suggest that pathways that recruit stress-activated protein/c-Jun NH2-terminal kinases may be activated. If confirmed, such findings suggest that the placenta in these pregnancies may have been exposed to a chronic inflammatory environment.

Finally, inflammation associated with GDM may persist beyond pregnancy and is a possible risk factor for the development of future inflammatory-related conditions. Heitritter and colleagues [57], using a case–control study, found that those who had GDM had significantly higher mean concentrations of inflammatory mediator, C-reactive protein, and lower concentrations of anti-inflammatory mediator, adiponectin, at approximately 4 years postpartum. These differences were maintained after adjusting for BMI.

## Immunomodulation and improved glucose metabolism

Pharmacologic inhibition of inflammatory mediators of the innate immune system has displayed promise in regard to improving glucose metabolism. Salicylates and thiazolidinediones exert anti-inflammatory effects and improve insulin sensitivity. Both classes of drugs have been shown to improve hyperglycemia. Salicylates exert their anti-inflammatory effects by inhibiting cycloxygenase production of prostaglandins, and also reduce inflammatory signaling by inhibition of nuclear factor-kappa B [58]. Nuclear factor-kappa B is a transcription factor, which, upon activation, induces gene expression of several inflammatory agents, inflammatory cytokines, as well as other genes that are involved in the inflammatory response. Nuclear factor-kappa B in its latent inactive form is bound by I-kappa kinase-beta, a group of inhibitory proteins, in the cytoplasm of most cell lines. Phosphorylation of I-kappa kinase-beta by IKK, a cellular kinase complex, leads to its degradation thereby allowing for the translocation of nuclear factor-kappa B into the nucleus where it activates genes that participate in the inflammatory process [59].

The effect of salicylates on glucose metabolism was confirmed by Hundal and colleagues [60] who gave aspirin, in high doses (6.2 gm/d), for 2 weeks to obese subjects who had T2DM. Upon completion of the 2-week trial period, they observed reduced fasting hyperglycemia, reduced basal hepatic glucose production, improved peripheral glucose uptake, and a 17% decrease in C-reactive protein concentration.

Thiazolidinediones are used clinically to increase insulin sensitivity. This class of agents binds to and activates peroxisome proliferator-activated receptors, which, like nuclear factor-kappa B, are transcription factors that regulate the expression of gene products important for adipocyte differentiation, fatty acid metabolism, glucose metabolism, and inflammation [61]. Peroxisome proliferator-activated receptors are found in adipocytes, pancreatic beta cells, vascular endothelium, macrophages, hepatocytes, cardiac muscle cells, skeletal muscle cells, and vascular walls. The diversity in cell types in which peroxisome proliferator-activated receptors are found contribute to the difficulty of ascribing one specific mechanism by which thiazolidinediones accomplish their insulin-sensitizing effects. The rise in insulin sensitivity may require the interaction of several cell types. The thiazolidinediones' anti-inflammatory effects result from the drug's stimulation of peroxisome proliferator-activated receptor-gamma in immune cells (monocytes), which inhibits their ability to produce inflammatory cytokines, such as TNF-α and interleukin-6 [62]. Clinically, thiazolidinediones have been associated with increased plasma concentrations of adiponectin; the potent anti-inflammatory adipokine [63]; as well as decreased serum concentrations of C-reactive protein [64], an acute phase reactant and general marker of inflammation.

## Summary

In summary, GDM likely reflects a chronic derangement of carbohydrate metabolism contributing to insulin resistance that is unmasked by a reduced ability of the pancreatic beta-cell to compensate for a pregnancy-induced further decline in insulin sensitivity. The pathophysiology of the chronic insulin resistance in these gravidas is likely due to obesity-related metabolic and immune dysregulation, both of which influence glycemic homeostasis by way of inflammatory mediators.

## References

[1] Kirwan JP, Hauguel-De Mouzon S, Lepercq J, et al. TNF-α is a predictor of insulin resistance in human pregnancy. Diabetes 2002;51:2207–13.

[2] Mills Jl, Jovanovic L, Knopp R, et al. Physiological reduction in fasting plasma glucose concentration in the first trimester of normal pregnancy: the diabetes in early pregnancy study. Metabolism 1998;47(9):1140–4.

[3] Catalano PM, Tyzbir ED, Wolfe RR, et al. Carbohydrate metabolism during pregnancy in control subjects and women with gestational diabetes. Am J Physiol Endocrinol Metab 1993; 264:E60–7.

[4] Catalano PM, Tyzibir ED, Roman NM, et al. Longitudinal changes in insulin resistance in non-obese pregnant women. Am J Obstet Gynecol 1991;165:1667–72.

[5] Sivan E, Chen XC, Homko CJ, et al. A longitudinal study of carbohydrate metabolism in healthy, obese pregnant women. Diabetes Care 1997;20(9):1470–5.

[6] American College of Obstetricians and Gynecologists Practice Bulletin. Clinical management guidelines for obstetricians-gynecologists. No. 30. September 2001. Obstet Gynecol 2001;98(3):525–38.

[7] Xiang AH, Peters RK, Trigo E, et al. Multiple metabolic defects during late pregnancy in women at high risk for type 2 diabetes. Diabetes 1999;48:848–54.

[8] Catalano PM, Huston L, Amini SB, et al. Longitudinal changes in glucose metabolism dur-
    ing pregnancy in obese women with normal glucose tolerance and gestational diabetes mel-
    litus. Am J Obstet Gynecol 1999;180(4):903–16.
[9] Buchanan TA, Xiang AH. Gestational diabetes. J Clin Invest 2005;115:485–91.
[10] Callaway LK, Prins JB, Chang AM, et al. The prevalence and impact of overweight and obe-
    sity in an Australian population. Med J Aust 2006;184(2):56–9.
[11] Friedman JE, Ishizuka T, Shao J, et al. Impaired glucose transport and insulin receptor ty-
    rosine phosphorylation in skeletal muscle and obsess women with gestational diabetes. Di-
    abetes 1999;48:1807–14.
[12] Homko C, Sivan E, Chen X, et al. Insulin secretion during and after pregnancy in patients
    with gestational diabetes mellitus. J Clin Endocrinol Metab 2001;86(2):568–73.
[13] Butler AE, Janson J, Bonner-Wier S, et al. Beta-cell deficit and increased beta-cell apoptosis
    in humans with type 2 diabetes. Diabetes 2003;52:102–10.
[14] Buchanan TA, Xiang AH, Peters RK, et al. Preservation of pancreatic beta cell function and
    prevention of type 2 diabetes by pharmacological treatment of insulin resistance in high-risk
    Hispanic women. Diabetes 2002;51:2796–803.
[15] Xiang AH, Peters RK, Kjos SL, et al. Effect of pioglitazone on pancreatic beta-cell function
    and diabetes risk in Hispanic women with prior gestational diabetes. Diabetes 2006;55:
    517–22.
[16] Fasshauer M, Kralisch S, Kiler M, et al. Insulin resistance-inducing cytokines differentially
    regulate SOCS mRNA expression via growth factor-X and Jak/Stat-signaling pathways in
    3T3-L1 adipocytes. J Endocrinol 2004;181:129–38.
[17] Rui L, Aguirre V, Dim JK, et al. Insulin/IGF-1 and TNF-a stimulate phosphorylation of
    IRS-1 at inhibitory Ser307 via distinct pathways. J Clin Invest 2001;107(2):181–9.
[18] Heinrich PC, Behrmann I, Muller-Newen G, et al. Interleukin-6-type cytokine signaling
    through the gp103/Jak/STAT pathway. Biochem J 1998;334:297–314.
[19] Heinrich PC, Behrmann I, Haan S, et al. Principles of interleukin (IL)-6-type cytokine sig-
    naling and its regulation. Biochem J 2003;374:1–20.
[20] Ogden CL, Carroll MD, Curtin LR, et al. Prevalence of overweight and obesity in the United
    States, 1999–2004. JAMA 2006;288(14):1723–7.
[21] Bianco AT, Smilen SW, Davis Y, et al. Pregnancy outcome and weight gain recommenda-
    tions for the morbidly obese woman. Obstet Gynecol 1998;91(1):97–102.
[22] Seibire N, Jolly M, Harris J, et al. Maternal obesity and pregnancy outcome: a study of
    287,213 pregnancies in London. Int J Obes 2001;25:1175–82.
[23] Kumari A. Pregnancy outcome on women with morbid obesity. Int J Gynaecol Obstet 2001;
    73(2):101–7.
[24] Baeten JM, Bukusi EA, Lambe M. Pregnancy complications and outcomes among over-
    weight and obese nulliparous women. Am J Public Health 2001;91:436–40.
[25] Boney CM, Verma A, Tucker R, et al. Metabolic syndrome in childhood: association with
    birth weight, maternal obesity, and gestational diabetes mellitus. Pediatrics 2005;115(3):
    e290–6.
[26] Charriere G, Cousin B, Arnaud E, et al. Preadipocyte conversion to macrophage. J Biol
    Chem 2003;278(11):9850–5.
[27] Kern PA, Di Gregorio GB, Lu T, et al. Adiponectin expression from human adipose tissue:
    relation to obesity, insulin resistance, and tumor necrosis factor-alpha expression. Diabetes
    2003;52:1779–85.
[28] Green A, Dobias SB, Walters DJ, et al. Tumor necrosis factor increases the rate of lipolysis in
    primary cultures of adipocytes without altering levels of hormone-sensitive lipase. Endocri-
    nology 1994;134(6):2581–8.
[29] Hotamisligil GS, Shargill NS, Spiegelman BM. Adipose expression of tumor necrosis factor-
    alpha: direct role in obesity-linked insulin resistance. Science 1993;259:87–91.
[30] Paresh D, Weinstock R, Thusu KE, et al. Tumor necrosis factor-α in sera of obese patients.
    Fall with weight loss. J Clin Endocrinol Metab 1998;83(8):2907–10.

[31] Hotamisligil GS, Arner P, Caro JF, et al. Increased adipose tissue expression of tumor necrosis factor-alpha in human obesity and insulin resistance. J Clin Invest 1995;95(5):2409–15.

[32] Heinrich PC, Castell JV, Andus T. Interleukin-6 and the acute phase response. Biochem J 1990;265(3):621–36.

[33] Bastard JP, Jardel C, Bruckert E, et al. Elevated levels of interleukin 6 are reduced in serum and subcutaneous adipose tissue of obese women after weight loss. J Clin Endocrinol Metab 2000;85(9):3338–42.

[34] Esposito K, Pontillo A, Di Palo C, et al. Effect of weight loss and lifestyle changes on vascular inflammatory markers in obese women: a randomized trial. JAMA 2003;289(14):1799–804.

[35] Tsigos C, Papanicolaou DA, Kyrou I, et al. Dose-dependent effects of recombinant human interleukin-6 on glucose regulation. J Clin Endocrinol Metab 1997;82:4167–70.

[36] Pittas AG, Joseph NA, Greenberg AS. Adipocytokines and insulin resistance. J Clin Endocrinol Metab 2004;89:447–52.

[37] Yokota T, Oritani K, Takahashi I, et al. Adiponectin, a new member of the family of soluble defense collagens, negatively regulates the growth of myelomonocytic progenitors and the function of macrophages. Blood 2000;96(5):1723–32.

[38] Statnick MA, Beavers LS, Conner LJ, et al. Decreased expression of apM1 in omental and subcutaneous adipose tissue of humans with type 2 diabetes. Int J Exp Diabetes Res 2000;1:81–8.

[39] Weyer C, Funahashi I, Tanaka S, et al. Hypoadiponectinemia in obesity and type 2 diabetes: close association with insulin resistance and hyperinsulinemia. J Clin Endocrinol Metab 2001;86:1930–5.

[40] Yang WS, Lee WJ, Funahashi T, et al. Weight reduction increases plasma levels of an adipose-derived anti-inflammatory protein, adiponectin. J Clin Endocrinol Metab 2001;86:3815–9.

[41] Yamauchi T, Kamon J, Waki H, et al. The fat-derived hormone adiponectin reverses insulin resistance associated with both lipoatrophy and obesity. Nat Med 2001;7:941–6.

[42] Sacks G, Sargent IL, Redman C. An innate view of human pregnancy. Immunol Today 1999;20:114–8.

[43] Sacks G, Studena K, Sargent IL, et al. Normal pregnancy and preeclampsia both produce inflammatory changes in peripheral leukocytes akin to those in sepsis. Am J Obstet Gynecol 1998;179(1):80–6.

[44] Belo L, Santos-Silva A, Rocha S, et al. Fluctuations in C-reactive protein concentration and neutrophil activation during normal human pregnancy. Eur J Obstet Gynecol Reprod Biol 2005;123:46–51.

[45] Richani K, Soto E, Romero R, et al. Normal pregnancy is characterized by systemic activation of the complement system. J Matern Fetal Neonatal Med 2005;17(4):239–45.

[46] Hunt JS, Robertson SA. Uterine macrophages and environmental programming for pregnancy success. J Reprod Immunol 1996;32(1):1–25.

[47] Jiang SP, Vacchio MS. Multiple mechanisms of peripheral T cell tolerance to the fetal "allograft". J Immunol 1998;161:2677–83.

[48] Wolf M, Sauk J, Shah A, et al. Inflammation and glucose intolerance: a prospective study of gestational diabetes mellitus. Diabetes Care 2004;27(1):21–7.

[49] Vozarova B, Weyer C, Tataranni PA, et al. High white blood cell count is associated with a worsening insulin sensitivity and predicts development of type 2 diabetes. Diabetes 2002;51:455–61.

[50] Schmidt MI, Duncan BB, Sharrett AR, et al. Markers of inflammation and prediction of diabetes mellitus in adults (atherosclerosis risk in communities studies): a cohort study. Lancet 1999;353:1649–52.

[51] Ategbo JM, Grissa O, Yessoufou A, et al. Modulation of adipokines and cytokines in gestational diabetes and macrosomia. J Clin Endocrinol Metab 2006;91(10):4137–43.

[52] Williams MA, Qiu C, Muy-Rivera M, et al. Plasma adiponectin concentration in early preg-
     nancy and subsequent risk of gestational diabetes mellitus. J Clin Endocrinol Metab 2004;
     89(5):2306–11.
[53] Richardson A, Fulton C, Catlow D, et al. Cytokine profiles in pregnant women with gesta-
     tional diabetes mellitus [abstract]. Am J Obstet Gynecol 2006;195(6):535.
[54] Esposito K, Pontillo A, Giugliano F. Association of low interleukin-10 levels with the met-
     abolic syndrome in obese women. J Clin Endocrinol Metab 2003;88(3):1055–8.
[55] Van Excel E, Gussekloo J, de Craen AJ. Low production capacity of interleukin-10 associ-
     ates with the metabolic syndrome and type 2 diabetes: The Leiden 85-plus study. Diabetes
     2002;51:1088–92.
[56] Radaelli T, Varastehpour A, Catalano P, et al. Gestational diabetes induces placental genes
     for chronic stress and inflammatory pathways. Diabetes 2003;52:2951–8.
[57] Heitritter SM, Solomon CG, Mitchell GF, et al. Subclinical inflammation and vascular dys-
     function in women with previous gestational diabetes mellitus. J Clin Endocrinol Metab
     2005;90(7):3983–8.
[58] Kopp E, Ghosh S. Inhibition of NF-kB by sodium salicylate and aspirin. Science 1994;265:
     956–9.
[59] Yin M, Yamamoto Y, Gaynor R. The anti-inflammatory agents aspirin and salicylate inhibit
     the activity of IkB kinase-beta. Nature 1998;396(5):77–80.
[60] Hundal RS, Petersen KF, Mayerson AB, et al. Mechanism by which high-dose aspirin im-
     proves glucose metabolism in type 2 diabetes. J Clin Invest 2002;109(10):1321–6.
[61] Yki-Jarvinen H. Thiazolidinediones. N Engl J Med 2004;351:1106–18.
[62] Jiang C, Ting AT, Seed B. PPAR-gamma agonists inhibit production of monocyte inflam-
     matory cytokines. Nature 1998;391:82–6.
[63] Maeda N, Takahasi M, Kihara S, et al. PPAR gamma ligands increase expression and
     plasma concentrations of adiponectin, an adipose-derived protein. Diabetes 2001;50:2094–9.
[64] Haffner SM, Greenberg AS, Weston WM, et al. Effect of rosiglitazone treatment on nontra-
     ditional markers of cardiovascular disease in patients with type 2 diabetes mellitus. Circula-
     tion 2002;106:679–84.

Obstet Gynecol Clin N Am
34 (2007) 225–239

OBSTETRICS AND
GYNECOLOGY
CLINICS
OF NORTH AMERICA

# Periconceptional Care of Women with Diabetes Mellitus

Gustavo Leguizamón, MD[a], María L. Igarzabal, MD[a],
E. Albert Reece, MD, PhD, MBA[b],*

[a]Department of Obstetrics and Gynecology, Center for Medical Education and Clinical
Research (C.E.M.I.C.) University, Av. Galván 4102, Buenos Aires, Argentina
[b]School of Medicine, University of Maryland, 655 W. Baltimore Street,
Room 14-029, Baltimore, Maryland 21201, USA

Diabetes mellitus (DM) is a metabolic disorder resulting from defects of insulin secretion or action, or both, leading to abnormalities in carbohydrate, protein, and lipid metabolism. Three types of DM have been classified: type 1, type 2, and gestational diabetes mellitus (occurring during pregnancy) [1]. This entity is one of the most common medical complications of pregnancy, with an incidence of 3% to 4% [2]. There are two groups of diabetic pregnant women: women with pregestational diabetes and women who develop diabetes during pregnancy (gestational diabetes). Because most women with pregestational diabetes receive no preconception care [3,4], they are exposed to high perinatal risks secondary to hyperglycemia and maternal vasculopathy. Diabetic women at childbearing ages face the following challenges: increase in major congenital malformations of their offspring, spontaneous abortion, and lack of information to make educated choices regarding potential progression of diabetic complications. The present article reviews current knowledge regarding the effect of pregestational diabetes on pregnancy outcomes as well as the impact of pregnancy on the progression of diabetes. The timing and type of interventions in preconception care to prevent pregnancy and maternal complications in diabetic women are also discussed.

* Corresponding author. Departments of Obstetrics and Gynecology and Biochemistry and Molecular Biology, 4301 West Markham Street, SLOT 550, Little Rock, AR 72205.
 E-mail address: deanmed@som.umaryland.edu (E.A. Reece).

0889-8545/07/$ - see front matter © 2007 Published by Elsevier Inc.
doi:10.1016/j.ogc.2007.04.002

**Major congenital anomalies**

*Significance*

In 1885, Le Corche [5] described, for the first time, the association between diabetes complicating pregnancy and congenital malformations. Pedersen [6] demonstrated that diabetic mothers were at high risk for birth defects. Since then, different types of malformations have been reported in infants born to diabetic women, with an estimated incidence of 6% to 10% [2]. The most commonly affected systems are cardiovascular, central nervous, gastrointestinal, genitourinary, and skeletal (Box 1) [7]. However, there is no specific diabetes-related anomaly. Sacral dysgenesis [8] and femoral hypoplasia–unusual facies phenotype [9] are the two exceptions. Only a small percentage of women with diabetes have children with these two defects.

---

**Box 1. Congenital anomalies commonly seen in infants of diabetic mothers**

Skeletal and central nervous system
Caudal regression syndrome
Neural tube defects excluding anencephaly
Anencephaly with or without herniation of neural elements
Microcephaly
Cardiac
Transposition of the great vessels with or without ventricular septal defects
Ventricular septal defects
Coarctation of the aorta with or without ventricular septal defects or patent ductus arteriosus
Atrial septal defects
Cardiomegaly
Renal anomalies
Hydronephrosis
Renal agenesis
Ureteral duplication
Gastrointestinal
Duodenal atresia
Anorectal atresia
Small left colon syndrome

---

*Data from* Reece EA, Hobbins JC. Diabetic embryopathy: pathogenesis, prenatal diagnosis and prevention. Obstet Gynecol Surv 1986;41:325.

The discovery of insulin in 1922 has changed the prognosis of patients affected by diabetes, including reproductive and pregnancy outcomes [10]. The following decades brought improvements in the management of pregnancies complicated by diabetes (eg, improved types of insulin and prenatal care), resulting in a dramatic reduction in maternal and perinatal morbidity and mortality [11]. In spite of these advancements, the rate of congenital malformations in the offspring of diabetic mothers remains high. Most studies observe a three- to fivefold increase in the rate of lethal congenital anomalies [6,12,13]. Congenital malformations account for almost 50% of the perinatal mortality for children born to diabetic mothers [14]; thus, identification of teratogens will lead to the development of targeted prevention programs. Although hyperglycemia has been shown to be teratogenic for the developing embryo, the intimate mechanism involved in maternal diabetes–induced dysmorphogenesis is not completely understood [15–18]. Hyperglycemia alone does not offer a complete explanation to the teratogenic process. Other factors such as myo-inositol and arachidonic acid deficiency [19], hyperketonemia [20], and excess of free oxygen radicals [21] were linked to birth defects in diabetic pregnancies in experimental and clinical models. Recent evidence demonstrated that hyperglycemia altered gene expression leading to aberrant cell signaling and resultant embryopathy [22]. These findings indicate that diabetic embryopathy may have a multifactorial etiology. Preconception counseling and care for diabetic women is the most important and effective intervention to reduce the incidence of congenital abnormalities in offspring.

## Effectiveness of preconception care in reducing the incidence of congenital malformations

Numerous studies have evaluated the outcome of pregnancy in diabetic women with intensified glycemic control during the preconception period and the first trimester of pregnancy. The notion that hyperglycemia during the period of organogenesis is a critical factor for the induction of congenital malformations, prompts investigators to test the effectiveness of preconception interventions on achieving and maintaining euglycemia.

From 1977 to 1981, Fuhrmann and colleagues [23] studied 420 women with insulin-dependent diabetes who delivered at the Department of Obstetrics and Gynecology of the Central Institute of Diabetes in Karlsburg, Germany. A group of 128 patients was admitted to the hospital every 3 months until conception and once more after pregnancy to attain glycemic control (60 to 130 mg/dL). Another group of 292 diabetic women began metabolic control after 8 weeks of conception. The former group showed 0.8% malformations and the second group showed 7.5%. The authors concluded that strict metabolic control in the periconceptional period reduces the rate of malformations in children of diabetic mothers.

Similar findings have been described by Steel and colleagues [24], who reported a 14-year experience of a prepregnancy clinic for diabetic women. There were 143 diabetic women who received prepregnancy care and 96 diabetic women who were in the control group. The study demonstrated lower hemoglobin A1c (HbA1c) concentration in the first trimester and lower rates of congenital malformations (1.4%) in the prepregnancy care group than in the control group (10.5%).

The Maine Diabetes Control Project [25], a statewide initiative with educational activities, was begun in 1985. There were 185 pregnancies from 160 women. In 34% of pregnancies, women with pregestational diabetes who received preconception counseling had 1.6% malformations while 66 pregnancies from diabetic women without preconception care yielded 6.5% malformations. Recently, by using a meta-analysis, Rey and colleagues [26] assessed the effect of preconception care on the occurrence of congenital malformations in 14 cohort studies involving 1192 offspring born by diabetic women who received preconception care and 1459 from diabetic women without such intervention. Preconception care decreased the rate of congenital anomalies from 6.5% to 2.1% (relative risk [RR] 0.36, 95% confidence interval [CI] 0.17-0.59). Other studies have reached similar results (Table 1) [23–25,27–35].

These reports support the hypothesis that achieving normoglycemia before and after conception reduces the rate of fetal anomalies.

Table 1
Incidence of major congenital anomalies in diabetic women with and without preconception care

| Clinical trials | IDDM with preconception care | | IDDM without preconception care | |
|---|---|---|---|---|
| | Number of infants | Congenital anomalies, n (%) | Number of infants | Congenital anomalies, n (%) |
| Fuhrmann et al [23] | 128 | 1 (0.8) | 292 | 16 (5.5) |
| Fuhrmann et al [31] | 56 | 1 (1.8) | 144 | 6 (4.2) |
| Goldman et al [27] | 44 | 0 | 31 | 2 (6.5) |
| Mills et al [32] | 347 | 17 (84.9) | 279 | 25 (9.0) |
| Damm and Molsted-Pedersen [33] | 283 | 7 (2.5) | 148 | 15 (10.1) |
| Steel et al [24] | 196 | 3 (81.5) | 117 | 14 (12.0) |
| Kitzmiller et al [30] | 84 | 1 (1.2) | 110 | 12 (10.9) |
| Rosenn et al [34] | 28 | 0 | 71 | 1 (1.4) |
| Tchobroutsky et al [35] | 40 | 0 | 186 | 16 (8.6) |
| Willhoite et al [25] | 58 | 1 (1.7) | 93 | 8 (8.6) |
| McElvy et al [28] | 92 | 2 (2.2) | 79 | 11 (14) |
| Evers et al [29] | 262 | 11 (4.2) | 49 | 6 (12.2) |

*Abbreviation:* IDDM, insulin dependent diabetes mellitus.

Because most pregnancies of diabetic women are either unplanned or without prenatal care until organogenesis has occurred, the efficacy of the intervention has been limited. In this context, education combined with accessibility to preconception care is the cornerstone of care in diabetic women and their infants.

## Maternal vasculopathy

### Nephropathy

Nephropathy complicates about 30% of women with type 1 DM. Overt nephropathy is defined as persistent proteinuria (more than 500 mg/ 24 hours of total protein or more than 300 mg/24 hours of urinary albumin excretion) observed in the first 20 weeks of pregnancy in the absence of urinary tract infection [36]. This condition is significantly correlated with the occurrence of maternal and fetal complications. Chronic hypertension and preeclampsia are observed in 40% of these subjects, retinopathy is present in 60%, and cesarean section is performed in over 70% of these women [37]. Perinatal complications are also significantly increased in this population. Preterm delivery occurs in 25% and intrauterine growth restriction (IUGR) in 15% of these pregnancies with an overall perinatal mortality rate of 5% [37]. Overall, pregnancy course tends to present more frequent and severe complications in women with nephropathy or moderate to severe renal function deterioration.

### Does pregnancy accelerate the progression of renal disease?

Studies addressing the short- and long-term impacts of pregnancy on renal function have limitations since they are retrospective and generally involve small groups of subjects and patients under different management strategies.

Many factors in pregnancy, such as chronic hypertension and superimposed preeclampsia, could have a significant impact on renal function. The physiologic increase in glomerular filtration rate (GFR) from 50% to 100% can also have a negative impact on kidney function. Several studies have addressed the changes in renovascular parameters throughout pregnancy in women with class F diabetes [37]. Proteinuria increases consistently from the first to the third trimester, returns to near prepregnancy levels at postpartum, and progresses at a similar rate to the natural history of diabetic nephropathy. Serum creatinine throughout pregnancy was found to be fairly stable if mild renal dysfunction was present preconceptionally. Patients with moderate to severe renal insufficiency in the first trimester demonstrate a more profound increase in serum creatinine toward the third trimester. Creatinine clearance did not show significant changes throughout pregnancy in the majority of the studies [37].

Long-term impact of pregnancy on progression of renal disease may be the most challenging issue when counseling patients with diabetic nephropathy who consider pregnancy. Kitzmiller and colleagues [38] reported renal function in 23 patients at 6 and 35 months postpartum. Proteinuria declined by 50% in 14 subjects, did not change in 7, and increased in only 2. No significant rise in serum creatinine was observed in the majority of the patients. Reece and colleagues [39] evaluated the rate of decline in renal function in 11 pregnancies with diabetic nephropathy. Mean serum creatinine measured within 4 years before conception, throughout pregnancy, and within 4 years after delivery did not differ from the expected decline observed in the absence of pregnancy. Miodovnik and colleagues [40] investigated whether pregnancy and parity could increase the risk for the development of nephropathy or accelerate the progression of preestablished renal disease among individuals with type I diabetes. The authors concluded that pregnancy did not increase the risk of development or progression of renal disease. These data indicate that pregnancy per se does not seem to hasten the progression of nephropathy to end-stage renal disease (ESRD); however, it must be interpreted with caution since most of the studies evaluated women with mild renal impairment. Studies discriminating women with nephropathy and moderate to severe renal impairment from those with normal or mild deterioration of renal function, showed different impact of pregnancy at follow-up. Several authors have supported this observation. Kimmerle and colleagues [41] evaluated 33 women with class F diabetes at 0.3 to 5 years postpartum. The authors reported a greater probability of requiring dialysis among 10 women with elevated serum creatinine at the beginning of the pregnancy than those with normal values. Furthermore, the rate of fall of creatinine clearance was minimal in women with normal Cr/Cl before pregnancy while those with preconception abnormal creatinine clearance showed greater fall. Purdy and colleagues [42] evaluated long-term outcomes in 11 patients with class F diabetes and moderate to severe renal impairment. These patients were compared with nonpregnant subjects with type 1 insulin-dependent DM (IDDM) and similar degrees of renal dysfunction. The authors concluded that patients with diabetic nephropathy and moderate to severe renal insufficiency had a 40% higher chance of accelerated progression of renal disease attributable to pregnancy effect. Finally, Gordon and colleagues [43] followed 34 subjects with class F diabetes for a mean period of 2.8 years. Patients with initial creatinine clearance greater than 90 mL/min and less than 1000 mg of protein in 24 hours had less progression of nephropathy. The authors concluded that renal function evaluation early in pregnancy can be helpful in predicting long-term progression of renal disease in pregnancy [10].

In summary, in patients with diabetic nephropathy and mild to moderate renal dysfunction (serum creatinine, 1.4 mg/dL and creatinine clearance over 90 mL/min), pregnancy per se does not worsen long-term outcome. On the other hand, pregnancy seems to accelerate renal function deterioration in women with moderate to severe renal dysfunction at the beginning of pregnancy.

*Proliferative retinopathy: class D and R diabetes*

Retinopathy is a common ocular complication of diabetes with a prevalence of 17% among patients diagnosed before age 30 with a disease duration of 5 years. After 15 years of diabetes, the prevalence rises to over 90% [44]. This is a progressive pathogenesis with two well-characterized stages: nonproliferative or background retinopathy (pregnancy Class D), and proliferative retinopathy (pregnancy Class R). The impact of pregnancy on the development or progression of proliferative retinopathy was studied by numerous investigators. Although some discrepancies exist beside methodological differences, it is clear that certain factors in pregnancy, such as duration of diabetes, degree of metabolic control, and hypertensive disorders, influence progression of proliferative retinopathy [45].

*Does pregnancy increase the development or progression of diabetic retinopathy?*

Most studies support the fact that pregnancy worsens diabetic retinopathy [45]. To assess the impact of pregnancy on retinopathy, a longitudinal analysis of the Diabetes Control and Complications Trial (DCCT) was performed [46]. This trial compared intensive therapy versus conventional therapy. The authors studied 180 women who had 270 pregnancies and 500 women who did not achieve any pregnancy during an average 6.5-year follow-up. Pregnant women in the intensive treatment group had 1.63-fold increased risk for worsening retinopathy during pregnancy when compared with nonpregnant subjects ($P < .05$). Those in the group of conventional therapy showed an increased risk of worsening retinopathy during pregnancy by 2.48-fold compared with nonpregnant women. Interestingly, this difference was transient and at the end of the follow-up period the authors observed no significant differences in retinopathy between pregnant and nonpregnant subjects.

For a woman seeking pregnancy, the risk of progression of retinopathy is clearly associated with the severity of preexisting disease. Rosenn and Miodovnik [2] observed that, in over 1000 pregnant women, the rate of developing to retinopathy during pregnancy in women without pregestational retinopathy, with pregestational background, and with proliferative retinopathy was 13%, 36%, and 43% respectively. Other factors consistently associated with progression of retinopathy are the degree of metabolic control as well as rapid normalization of glucose [45]. Chew and colleagues [47] conducted a prospective cohort study of 155 diabetic women in the Diabetes in Early Pregnancy Study. The authors observed significant association between elevated HbA1c at baseline or the magnitude of improvement of early metabolic control and progression of retinopathy. Since these two factors are usually interrelated, it is difficult to determine if these effects are independent.

Finally, hypertensive disorders during pregnancy have also been linked to the progression of retinopathy. Rosenn and colleagues [48] prospectively followed 154 diabetic women. Evidence for retinopathy was determined during pregnancy and at 6 and 12 weeks postpartum. The authors found that both the presence of chronic hypertension and pregnancy-induced hypertension were significantly associated with progression of retinopathy.

Based on this evidence, preconception evaluation of the retinal status is of most importance since it allows detection and treatment of proliferative disease before conception. If retinopathy is present, a planned slow reduction of HbA1c should be achieved avoiding sudden glycemic changes. Finally, identification of risk factors for progression will prompt an intensive follow-up of retinal pathology during pregnancy.

## Coronary heart disease: class H diabetes

Although coronary artery disease (CAD) is uncommon among women in their reproductive years, type 1 DM increases the risk of myocardial infarction from 1 in 10,000 in the general population to 1 in 350 [49,50].

From 1953 to date, 24 cases of class H diabetes have been reported in the world's literature [51]. Maternal and fetal survival, timing and year of the coronary event, as well as presence of coronary artery bypass graft (CABG), are depicted in (Table 2). The analysis of these data is limited since the number of patients is small, and the available information on residual cardiac function is incomplete. With these limitations in mind, three general observations can be made:

(1) No maternal or fetal deaths occurred among patients who had a CABG before pregnancy while 38% maternal or fetal death occurred in those who did not receive such preconception care. The

Table 2
Maternal and fetal survival according to period of treatment and presence of coronary artery bypass graft (CABG) and timing of the event

|  | 1980 (overall) | | CABG | | Time of AMI relative to pregnancy | |
|---|---|---|---|---|---|---|
|  | Before | After | (−) | (+) | Before | During-after |
| Maternal mortality | 73% | 0% | 38% | 0% | 0% | 62% |
|  | (8/11) | (0/12) | (8/21) | (0/3) | (0/11) | (8/13) |
| Fetal loss | 50% | 0% | 30% | 0% | 9% | 42% |
|  | (5/10) | (0/12) | (6/20) | (0/3) | (1/11) | (5/12) |

*Abbreviation:* AMI, acute myocardial infarction.

*Data from* Leguizamón G, Reece EA. Diabetic neuropathy and coronary artery disease. In: Reece EA, Coustan DR, Gabbe SG, editors. Diabetes in women: adolescence, pregnancy, and menopause. 3rd edition. Philadelphia, PA: Lippincott Williams & Wilkins; 2004. p. 425–32.

benefit of a CABG performed before pregnancy in properly selected women seems to be supported, and is possibly related to the increased survival observed. The impact of this treatment is difficult to assess since these cases were reported after 1980 when the overall outcome was improved.

(2) Maternal mortality was extremely high (73%) among patients reported before 1980 with a dramatic improvement thereafter (no maternal deaths).

(3) There were no maternal deaths associated with preconception myocardial infarction (MI), but a mortality rate of 62% was observed when it occurred during pregnancy or the puerperium.

Preconceptional evaluation and possible treatment of CAD patients with a bypass graft may improve maternal and perinatal outcomes. Although further evidence is required, it appears that preconception correction of CAD may help to improve cardiac tolerance to the pregnant state with a subsequent prolongation of pregnancy and diminished morbidity from prematurity. Finally, the review of the recent literature on class H diabetes reveals that pregnancy does not appear to have as ominous a prognosis as was once reported. Nevertheless, given the fairly high maternal mortality rate, pregnancy should still be considered relatively contraindicated until further information confirms a more favorable trend.

*Neuropathy*

Diabetic neuropathy is a heterogeneous group of abnormalities involving both the autonomic and peripheral nervous systems. Somatic neuropathies include symmetrical distal polyneuropathy, cranial neuropathy, and radiculopathy or truncal mononeuropathy; while autonomic neuropathies include cardiovascular (resting tachycardia, exercise intolerance, and orthostatic hypotension), gastrointestinal (abnormal esophageal motility, gastroparesis, diarrhea, constipation), genitourinary (neurogenic bladder, sexual dysfunction), and hypoglycemia unawareness [51].

*Does pregnancy accelerate the progression or induce the occurrence of diabetic neuropathy among diabetic women?*

Early investigations suggested that pregnancy could enhance the progression of neuropathy [52]. That concept, however, was challenged by recent findings. In 1995, the EURODIAB type 1 complications study [53] compared the impact of parity among 1358 nonpregnant women with type 1 diabetes. The authors concluded that parity does not influence the long-term prevalence or severity of diabetic autonomic neuropathy. Hemachandra and colleagues [54] conducted two, nested, pair-matched case control studies to determine the short- and long-term impacts of parity on the prevalence of autonomic neuropathy. Patients were examined for the presence of distal sensory-motor neuropathy at baseline and 2 and 4 years after inclusion. In the first study, the prevalence of neuropathy in 80 diabetic women who achieved pregnancy was compared with that in women who remained nulligravid at 4-year follow-up. The authors concluded that the long-term (4 years) prevalence of distal symmetric polyneuropathy was not increased by parity. In the second study, the short-term effect (less than 2 years) was evaluated. Interestingly, the incidence of neuropathy was 10 times higher for parous women than for women in the nulliparous controls (41.7% versus 4.8%, odds ratio [OR] 10.00, confidence interval 1.10->100-). Therefore, these studies indicate that although pregnancy may accelerate the development of neuropathy in the short term, there is no evidence of poor prognosis in the long range. Finally, Lapolla and colleagues [55] addressed the issue of initial development of somatic and autonomic neuropathy. The patients were evaluated three times during pregnancy and once at 6-month follow-up. Controls consisted of one group of matched nonpregnant diabetic women, and another group of matched nondiabetic pregnant women to reduce potential bias secondary to the normal blunted autonomic response reported in uncomplicated pregnancies. The authors concluded that women with mild or no evidence of neuropathy are not affected by pregnancy. Interestingly, conduction velocities improved in pregnant diabetic women toward the third trimester. Because the DCCT trial demonstrated that tight glucose control significantly reduced disease progression [56], a possible explanation for this unexpected finding is the improved glycemic control achieved during pregnancy.

Therefore, current literature supports the notion that pregnancy is not a risk factor for the development or progression of either autonomic or somatic diabetic neuropathy.

## Does diabetic autonomic neuropathy affect pregnancy outcome?

Gastroparesis interferes with food absorption and is therefore associated with difficulties in blood glucose control and is commonly associated with severe nausea and vomiting. Because severe maternal and fetal morbidity have been reported in association with this condition, special consideration should be taken during the preconception period. Although its diagnosis is not well standardized, presence of a history of chronic nausea and vomiting compel to further evaluation. The finding of food in the stomach after 8 to 12 hours of fasting is sufficient for the diagnosis. Endoscopy also serves to rule out other causes of vomiting, and a detailed history regarding a pharmacological etiology is essential.

Analysis of maternal and fetal outcomes in pregnancies with gastroparesis reveals that perinatal mortality, congenital malformations, polyhydramnios, preterm delivery, preeclampsia, hypoglycemic episodes, and ketoacidosis, were increased up to twofold in patients with diabetic neuropathy than in control subjects [51].

The most worrisome aspect of diabetic autonomic neuropathy during pregnancy is the occurrence of gastroparesis diabeticorum. This entity may result in significant maternal and fetal morbidity. This condition, when severe, has been associated with significant maternal complications such as pulmonary edema or aspiration, the need for parenteral nutrition, and poor glucose control. Severe fetal complications such as intrauterine growth restriction (IUGR), preterm labor, and fetal loss [57] also have been reported. Severe gastroparesis complicating pregnancy is unusual and only a few cases have been reported in the world's literature [52,58–60].

Based on these serious complications, pregnancy could be considered a relative contraindication in patients with severe diabetic gastroparesis. Furthermore, the fact that autonomic function tests could be altered during pregnancy highlights the importance of preconception screening for gastroparesis allowing identification of more severe cases and proper counseling regarding potential maternal and perinatal morbidity and mortality.

### Guidelines for preconception care

The main objectives of preconception counseling for diabetic women are the following:

(1) Folic acid administration and adequate blood glucose control before conception decrease the rate of major congenital anomalies. Monitoring HbA1c levels monthly until stable at a level of less than 1% above the upper limit of normal. Patients should also be educated regarding contraceptive use throughout this period.

(2) Evaluation with history, physical examination, and laboratory determinations for presence of diabetic-related complications:

*Diabetic nephropathy:* 24-hour urine collection to determine if proteinuria is present. Also creatinine clearance, serum creatinine, and BUN should be determined. Furthermore, urinary cultures should be obtained.

*Diabetic retinopathy:* dilated retinal exam by an ophthalmologist is indicated. In case of retinopathy, background versus proliferative must be noted.

*Cardiovascular system:* determination of blood pressure is of outmost importance in this population. If chronic hypertension was previously diagnosed, a review of antihypertensive medications should be performed. If ACE inhibitors are being used, they should be replaced by less embryotoxic treatment. An EKG should be obtained in women with 10 or more years of diabetes, hypertension, or other evidence of vasculopathy. Any suspicion of CAD should be further evaluated with an exercise stress test.

*Evidence of autonomic dysfunction* such as lack of awareness of hypoglycemia and orthostatic hypotension, as well as excessive nausea

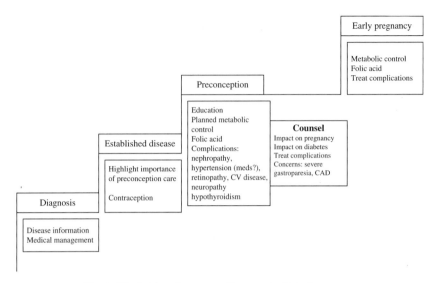

Fig. 1. The ladder of preconception care in diabetic women.

and vomiting should prompt further evaluation of these diabetic complications.

*Endocrine:* since thyroid dysfunction is frequently associated with type 1 diabetes, thyroid function should be routinely evaluated in the preconception period (Fig. 1).

## Summary

Pregestational diabetes is a common complication of pregnancy that can be associated with severe maternal and fetal morbidity. In addition, some women could have progression of diabetic complications secondary to pregnancy. Preconception care can significantly reduce pregnancy complications with a dramatic impact on the diabetic mother and her infant. For those women whose condition could be hastened by conception education, better understanding and an improved decision should be available to them and their families. Because unplanned pregnancy is common among diabetic women, they should be counseled early for the importance of preconception care in the progression of this disease.

## References

[1] American Diabetes Association. Position statement. Diagnosis and classification of diabetes mellitus. American Diabetes Association Diabetes Care 2007;30(Suppl 1):S42–7.
[2] Rosenn BM, Miodovnik M. Preconceptional care of women with diabetes. In: Reece EA, Coustan DR, Gabbe SG, editors. Diabetes in women adolescence, pregnancy, and menopause. 3rd edition. Philadelphia, PA: Lippincott Williams & Wilkins; 2004. p. 73–90.

[3] American Diabetes Association. Position statement. Preconception care of women with diabetes. Diabetes Care 2003;26(Suppl 1).

[4] Suhonen L. Glycemic control during early pregnancy and fetal malformations in women with type I diabetes mellitus. Diabetologia 2000;43(1):79–82.

[5] Le Corche E. Du Diabetic dans ses rapports avec la vie uterine menstruation, et al grusesse. Annales de Gynecologic 1885;24:257.

[6] Pedersen J. The pregnant diabetic and her newborn. 2nd edition. Baltimore (MD): Williams & Wilkins; 1977.

[7] Reece EA, Hobbins JC. Diabetic embryopathy: pathogenesis, prenatal diagnosis and prevention. Obstet Gynecol Surv 1986 Jun;41(6):325–35, Review.

[8] Welch JP, Aterman K. The syndrome of caudal dysplasia: a review, including etiologic considerations and evidence of heterogeneity. Pediatr Pathol 1984;2:313–27.

[9] Hurst D, Johnson DF. Brief clinical report: femoral hypoplasia-unusual facies syndrome. Am J Med Genet 1980;5:255–8.

[10] Banting FG, Best CH. The internal secretion of the pancreas. Best CH Can Med Assoc J 1962 Nov 17;87:1046–51.

[11] Jovanovic L, Peterson CM. Management of the pregnant, insulin-dependent diabetic women. Diabetes Care 1980;6:63–8.

[12] Kucera J. Rate and type of congenital anomalies among offspring of diabetic women. J Reprod Med 1971;7(2):73–83.

[13] Drury MI, Greene AT, Stronge JM. Pregnancy complicated by clinical diabetes mellitus. A study of 600 pregnancies Obstet Gynecol 1977 May;49(5):519–22.

[14] Hadden DR, Traub AI, Harley JMG. Diabetes-related perinatal mortality and congenital fetal abnormality: a problem of audit. Diabet Med 1988;5:321–3.

[15] Endo A. Teratogenesis in diabetic mice treated with alloxan prior to conception. Arch Environ Health 1966;12:492–500.

[16] Cockroft DI, Coppola PT. Teratogenic effects of excess glucose on head-fold rat embryos in culture. Teratology 1977;16:141–6.

[17] Sadler TW. Effects of maternal diabetes on early embryogenesis II. Hyperglycemia induced exencephaly. Teratology 1980 Jun;21(3):349–56.

[18] Reece EA, Pinter E, Leranth CZ, et al. Ultrastructural analysis of malformations of the embryonic neural axis induced by in vitro hyperglycemic conditions. Teratology 1985;32: 363–72.

[19] Hod M, Star S, Passonnequ JV, et al. Effect of hyperglycemia on sorbitol and myoinositol content of cultured rat conceptus: failure of aldose reductase inhibitors to midify myo-inositol depletion and dysmorphogenesis. Biochem Biophys Res Commun 1986; 140:974–80.

[20] Horton WE, Sadler TW, Hunter ES. Effects of hyperketonemia on mouse embryonic and fetal glucose metabolism in vitro. Teratology 1985;31:227–33.

[21] Eriksson UJ, Borg LAH. Protection by free oxygen radical scavenging enzymes against glucose-induced embryonic malformations in vitro. Diabetologia 1991;34:325–31.

[22] Reece EA, Ji I, Wu YK, et al. Characterization of differential gene expression profiles in diabetic embryopathy using DNA microarray analysis. Am J Obstet Gynecol 2006;195(4): 1075–80.

[23] Fuhrmann K, Reiher H, Semmler K, et al. Prevention of congenital malformations in infants of insulin-dependent diabetic mothers. Diabetes Care 1983;6:219–23.

[24] Steel JM, Jhonstone FD, Hepburn, et al. Can pregnancy care of diabetic women reduce the risk of abnormal babies? BMJ 1990;301:1070–4.

[25] Willhoite MB, Bennert HW, Palomaki GE, et al. The impact of preconception counseling in pregnancy outcomes. The experience of the Maine Diabetes in Pregnancy Program. Diabetes Care 1993;16:450–5.

[26] Rey JG, O'Brien TE, Chan WS. Preconception care and the risk of congenital anomalies in the offspring of women with diabetes mellitus: a meta-analysis. QJM 2001;94(8):435–44.

[27] Goldman JA, Dicker D, Feldberg D, et al. Pregnancy outcome in patients with insulin-dependent diabetes mellitus with preconceptional diabetes control: a comparative study. Am J Obstet Gynecol 1986;155:293–7.

[28] McElvy SS, Miodovnik M, Rosenn B, et al. A focused preconceptional and early pregnancy program in women with type I diabetes reduces perinatal mortality and malformation rates to general population levels. J Matern Fetal Med 2000;9(1):14–20.

[29] Evers IM, deValk HW, Visser GH. Risk of complications of pregnancy in women with Type I diabetes: nationwide prospective study in the Netherlands. BMJ 2004 Apr 17; 328(7445):915. Equb 2004 Apr 5.

[30] Kitzmiller JL, Gavin LA, Gin GD, et al. Preconception management of diabetes continued through early pregnancy prevents the excess frequency of major congenital anomalies in infant of diabetic mother. JAMA 1991;265:731–6.

[31] Fuhrmann K, Reiher H, Semmler K, et al. The effect of intensified conventional insulin therapy before and during pregnancy on the malformation rate in offspring of diabetic mothers. Exp Clin Endocrinol 1984;83:173–7.

[32] Mills JL, Knopp RH, Simpson JL, et al. Lack of relation of increased malformation rates in infants of diabetic mothers to glycemic control during organogenesis. N Engl J Med 1988; 318(11):671–6.

[33] Damm P, Molsted-Pedersen L. Significant decrease in congenital malformations in newborn infants of an unselected population of diabetic women. Am J Obstet Gynecol 1989;161(5): 1163–7.

[34] Rosenn B, Miodovnik M, Combs CA, et al. Pre-conception management of insulin-dependent diabetes: improvement of pregnancy outcome. Obstet Gynecol 1991;77(6):846–9.

[35] Tchobroutsky C, Vray MM, Altman JJ. Risk/benefit ratio of changing late obstetrical strategies in the management of insulin-dependent diabetic pregnancies. A comparison between 1971–1977 and 1978–1985 periods in 389 pregnancies. Diabete Metab 1991;17(2):287–94.

[36] Kitzmiller JL. Diabetes in women: adolescence, pregnancy, and menopause. In: Reece EA, Coustan DR, Gabbe SG, editors. 3rd edition. Philadelphia, PA: Lippincott Williams & Wilkins; 2004. p. 382–423.

[37] Reece EA, Leguizamon G, Homko C. Pregnancy performance and outcomes associated with diabetic nephropathy. Am J Perinatol 1998 Jul;15(7):413–21, Review.

[38] Kitzmiller JL, Brown ER, Phillippe M, et al. Diabetic nephropathy and perinatal outcome. Am J Obstet Gynecol 1981 Dec 1;141(7):741–51.

[39] Reece EA, Winn HN, Hayslett JT, et al. Does pregnancy alter the rate of progression of diabetic nephropathy? Am J Perinatol 1990 Apr;7(2):193–7.

[40] Miodovnik M, Rosenn BM, Khoury JC, et al. Does pregnancy increase the risk for development and progression of diabetic nephropathy? Am J Obstet Gynecol 1996;174:1180–91.

[41] Kimmerle R, Zass R-P, et al. Pregnancies in women with diabetic nephropathy: Long-term outcome for mother and child. Diabetologia 1995 Feb;38(2):227–35.

[42] Purdy LP, Hantsch CE, Molitch ME, et al. Effect of pregnancy on renal function in patients with moderate-to-severe diabetic renal insufficiency. Diabetes Care 1996;19:1067–74.

[43] Gordon M, Landon M, Samuels P, et al. Perinatal outcome and long-term follow up associated with modern management of diabetic nephropathy. Obstet Gynecol 1996;87:401–9.

[44] Klein R, Klein BE, Moss S, et al. The Wisconsin epidemiologic study of diabetic retinopathy. IV. Diabetic macular edema. Ophthalmology 1984;91(12):1464–74.

[45] Sheth B. Does pregnancy accelerate the rate of progression of diabetic retinopathy? [review]. Curr Diab Rep 2002;2(4):327–30.

[46] The Diabetes Control and Complications Trial Research Group. Effect of pregnancy on microvascular complications in the diabetes control and complications trial. Diabetes Care 2000;23(8):1084–91.

[47] Chew EY, Mills JL, Metzger BE, et al. Metabolic control and progression of retinopathy. The Diabetes in Early Pregnancy Study. National Institute of Child Health and Human Development Diabetes in Early Pregnancy Study. Diabetes Care 1995;18(5):631–7.

[48] Rosenn B, Miodovnik M, Kranias G, et al. Progression of diabetic retinopathy in pregnancy: association with hypertension in pregnancy. Am J Obstet Gynecol 1992;166(4):1214–8.

[49] Fletcher E, Knox EW, Morton P. Acute myocardial infarction in pregnancy. Br Med J 1967 September 2;3(5565):586–8.

[50] Sullivan JM, Ramanathan KB. Management of medical problems in pregnancy—severe cardiac disease. N Engl J Med 1985;313:304.

[51] Leguizamón G, Reece EA. Diabetic neuropathy and coronary artery disease. In: Reece EA, Coustan DR, Gabbe SG, editors. Diabetes in women: adolescence, pregnancy, and menopause. 3rd edition. Philadelphia, PA: Lippincott Williams & Wilkins; 2004. p. 425–32.

[52] Macleod AF, Smith SA, Sonksen PH, et al. The problem of autonomic neuropathy in diabetic pregnancy. Diabet Med 1990 Jan;7(1):80–2.

[53] Chaturvedi N, Stephenson JM, Fuller JH, et al. The relationship between pregnancy and long-term maternal complications in the EURODIAB IDDM complications study. Diabet Med 1995;12:494–9.

[54] Hemachandra A, Ellis D, Lloyd K, et al. The influence of pregnancy on IDDM complications. Diabetes Care 1995;18(7):950–4.

[55] Airaksinen KEJ, Salmela PI, Markku J, et al. Effect of pregnancy on autonomic nervous function and heart rate in diabetic and nondiabetic women. Diabetes Care 1987;10:748–51.

[56] The Diabetes Control and Complications Trial Research Group. The effect of intensive treatment of diabetes on the development and progression of long-term complications in insulin-dependent diabetes mellitus. N Engl J Med 1993;329:977–86.

[57] Hagay Z, Weissman A. Management of diabetic pregnancy complicated by coronary artery disease and neuropathy. Obstet Gynecol Clin North Am 1996;23(1):205–20.

[58] Hare JW, White P. Pregnancy in diabetes complicated by vascular disease. Diabetes 1977 Oct;26(10):953–5.

[59] Steel JM. Autonomic neuropathy in pregnancy [letter]. Diabetes Care 1989;12:170–1.

[60] Guy RJC, Dawson JL, Garrett JT, et al. Diabetic gastroparesis from autonomic neuropathy: surgical considerations and changes in vagus nerve morphology. J Neurol Neurosurg Psychiatry 1984;47:686–91.

ELSEVIER
SAUNDERS

Obstet Gynecol Clin N Am
34 (2007) 241–253

OBSTETRICS AND
GYNECOLOGY
CLINICS
OF NORTH AMERICA

# Use of New Technologies for Monitoring and Treating Diabetes in Pregnancy

Yariv Yogev, MD*, Moshe Hod, MD

*Perinatal Division, Helen Schneider Hospital for Women, Rabin Medical Center,
Petach Tikva, 49100, Tel Aviv University, Israel*

In the United States, depending upon the diagnosis criteria used, 135 to 200,000 women annually develop gestational diabetes (GDM), adding to the number of pregnant women already suffering from either type 1 or type 2 diabetes. The maternal hyperglycemia and the resultant fetal hyperinsulinemia are central to the pathophysiology of diabetic complications of pregnancy. These complications include congenital malformations and an increase in neonatal intensive care unit admission and birth trauma. In addition, there is an increased rate of accelerated fetal growth, neonatal metabolic complications, and risk for stillbirth [1–4]. During the last century, there were two breakthroughs in diabetes management and monitoring that changed the course of treatment: the discovery of insulin and the progress in the understanding of glucose monitoring. As technology evolved, both glucose monitoring and insulin administration can now be achieved in a continuous fashion. In this review, the authors focus on the utility of new technologies in the management and monitoring of diabetes in pregnancy.

## Glucose monitoring during pregnancy:
### from glucosuria to continuous glucose monitoring

The ability to monitor glucose values is of historical significance; throughout recorded history, physicians have been familiar with diabetes and have "finger-dipped" to detect the "sweetness" of patients' urine. This imperfect technique was used until the development of urine sticks in the early twentieth century that were sensitive enough to detect glucosuria.

---

* Corresponding author.
*E-mail address:* yarivyogev@hotmail.com (Y. Yogev).

0889-8545/07/$ - see front matter © 2007 Elsevier Inc. All rights reserved.
doi:10.1016/j.ogc.2007.03.005               *obgyn.theclinics.com*

Research efforts have continuously been directed toward the development of a process for testing blood glucose using either visual or electronic interpretation with a reflectance meter. The method of testing that was developed was based on obtaining a sample of capillary blood with specially designed lancets and placing it on a test strip composed of glucose oxidase and peroxidase. The strips were visually read, went through a color change, and matched against a color chart that provided blood glucose ranges but not specific glucose values.

*A single measure of glycemic level: glycosylated hemoglobin and glycosylated protein*

Traditionally, in nonpregnant diabetic patients, glycosylated hemoglobin ($HbA_1$) became the predictor of long-term glycemia. $HbA_1$ is a modification of hemoglobin caused by the attachment of glucose to the N-terminus of the beta chain. The rate of attachment is determined by the glucose concentration in the blood. Based on the lifespan of the red blood cells, which averages 120 days, different reports have suggested that the predictability of $HbA_1$ ranges from 4 to 10 weeks [5–7]. In pregnancy, glycosylated hemoglobin does not correlate well with glycemic profile [8,9]. This is especially true in patients who have gestational diabetes whose blood glucose is mildly elevated in comparison to type 1 and type 2 diabetes patients. Studies have reported no to moderate correlations between $HbA_1$ and different components of the glucose profile when an $HbA_1$ result of 4% to 5% includes a capillary blood glucose range of 50 to 160 mg/dL. Some diabetic programs still use levels of glycosylated hemoglobin as a glycemic goal in the management of GDM. Levels of HbA1c are related to the rate of congenital anomalies and spontaneous early abortions in pre-existing diabetes, but the use of this measure, which retrospectively reflects glycemic profile in the last 10 weeks, for treatment evaluation in GDM is questionable. In addition, the association between glycosylated hemoglobin and pregnancy outcome in GDM or prediction of macrosomia is poor [10–13]. Furthermore, the lack of uniformity among different laboratories has resulted in multiple thresholds of normality obscuring HbA1c efficiency for routine use. Therefore, from the authors' point of view, using HbA1c as a tool for monitoring glycemic goal and treatment adjustment in managing GDM is not effective.

A second single measure is either glycosylated protein or fructosamine. Both have shorter life spans (7–10 days) and, therefore, may be used as a measure for short-term glucose profile evaluation. However, in pregnancy, a wide variability was found when they were compared with self-blood glucose measurements and, to date, their role in evaluation of level of glycemia has not yet been established.

*The use of self-blood glucose monitoring*

In the late twentieth century, it became technically achievable to test blood glucose values using reflectance meters. The original meters used a wet method that often required as many as four steps (approximately 10 minutes/ step) to obtain one test result. Today's reflectance meters are more user-friendly; they include a memory chip for data storage and one-step testing.

This technologic advancement made it possible for patients to monitor self-blood glucose measurements and test blood glucose values independent of care providers. Using this technology was the cornerstone in establishment of an *intensified management approach* for glycemic monitoring and control during pregnancy complicated by diabetes. Intensified therapy is an approach to achieving established levels of glycemic control. It incorporates memory-based self-monitoring blood glucose, multiple injections of insulin or its equivalent, diet, and an interdisciplinary team effort. It was demonstrated in a large prospective study that intensified therapy, in comparison to the conventional approach in women who have GDM, results in pregnancy outcome comparable to the general population [14]. Independent of the particular treatment modality used and the type of diabetes, memory-based self-monitoring blood glucose accurately quantifies the glucose data that sets the foundation for achieving success with intensified therapy. Capillary blood glucose monitoring provides the feedback for suitable adjustments to the timing and dose of insulin administration. Patients who have all types of diabetes readily acknowledge and accept self-monitoring blood glucose as an expression of patient empowerment because they are involved in the efforts to improve pregnancy outcome.

*Continuous glucose monitoring system*

Recently, several companies have attempted to develop a new technology that measures continuous glucose. Some of these techniques are noninvasive, and others are minimally invasive [15]. Glucose monitoring methods employ four different approaches: transdermal, glucose electrode, microdialysis, or open-flow microperfusion. Currently, two are commercially available. The transdermal approach (Glucowatch; Cygnus Inc., Redwood City, California) employs reverse iontophoresis by applying low-voltage current to the skin surface causing interstitial fluid (containing glucose) to pass through the skin. Glucose is then measured by an oxidase reaction. These data also contain information about skin temperature and sweat that are all included in the calculation process [16]. The MiniMed Continuous Glucose Monitoring (CGM) System (MiniMed, Inc., Sylmar, California) is composed of a disposable subcutaneous glucose-sensing device and an electrode impregnated with glucose oxidase connected by a cable to a lightweight monitor, which is worn over clothing or a belt. The system measures glucose levels every 10 seconds, based on the electrochemical detection of glucose by its reaction with glucose oxidase, and stores an average value every 5 minutes, for a total of 288 measurements per day. The glucose measurement is performed in subcutaneous tissue in which the interstitial glucose levels are in the range of 40 to 400 mg/dL. The data are stored in the monitor for later downloading and reviewing on a personal computer (Fig. 1). The patients are unaware of the results of the sensor measurements during the monitoring period. Glucose values obtained with CGM have been shown to correlate with laboratory measurements of plasma glucose levels [17] and with home glucose meter values [18]. To corroborate CGM system accuracy, patients are expected to perform three to five capillary blood tests daily using conventional meters. This additional chore becomes a potential burden for the patient.

*Glucose monitoring using continuous glucose monitoring system in nondiabetic pregnancy: understanding normal glycemic profile in pregnancy*

The goal of management in pregnancy complicated with diabetes is to maintain blood glucose as near to normal as possible. However, paucity of data exists concerning the normal glycemic profile in nondiabetic pregnancies [19–21]. Moreover, these studies included small sample sizes in a hospital environment under strict diet limitations; some of the patients were diabetic [19]. Data included only a single day of evaluation during the third trimester. Moreover, no stratification was performed for obesity. In a recent study [22], the maternal glycemic profile was evaluated using self-monitoring blood glucose in nonobese, nondiabetic women during the third trimester, suggesting a gradual increase in daily mean glucose during this time. Using CGM, the authors analyzed [23] 3 days of continuous glucose monitoring in nondiabetic gravid patients. During the study period, all women were asked

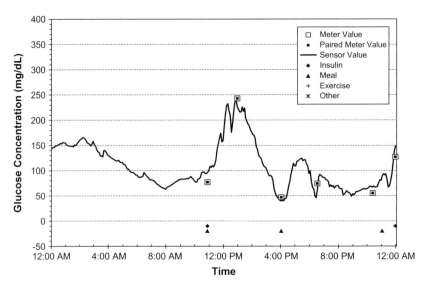

Fig. 1. Twenty-four–hour continuous glucose monitoring using continuous glucose monitoring system.

to refrain from lifestyle modification or dietary restriction. Patients were monitored for 72 consecutive hours and were unaware of the results of the sensor measurements during the monitoring period. During this period, they also performed finger stick capillary glucose measurements in the morning after overnight fasting and 2 hours after meals (6–8 times per day) using a reflectance monitor and self-coded the data into the monitor. Quality control measures of glucose levels from the meter, sensor, and plasma glucose were performed at the initial time of connection to the continuous glucose monitoring system and again at study completion. Approximately 750 glucose determinations were obtained for each subject during this time period. Thus, ambulatory glycemic profile during the second half of pregnancy was characterized enabling the authors to define normal glycemia (Table 1). When the authors further analyzed the ambulatory glycemic profile, they found no difference in preprandial values throughout the day and significantly lower mean blood glucose levels during the nighttime (23:00 PM–06:00 AM) in comparison to daytime (see Table 1). These findings are lower than some have previously reported [19,20] but in agreement with others [22]. Thus, the authors' data may provide the characterization of glycemic profile in the second half of pregnancy, which would inform the level of glycemia to be targeted to mirror normoglycemia in the pregnant diabetic. Whether normoglycemia should be targeted, and whether there are any dangers implicit in targeting normoglycemia for women who have GDM is a subject for future investigation.

## Postprandial glycemic profile: a hint for improved management?

By using continuous glucose monitoring, the authors evaluated postprandial glycemic profile in diabetic pregnancies [24]. They showed that the time interval from meal to peak postprandial glucose levels was approximately 90 minutes, a finding that was similar in all patients who had GDM unrelated to mode of treatment and was not affected by the level of glycemic control. This was somewhat later than the 70-minute peaks they observed in

Table 1
Ambulatory glycemic profile in nondiabetic pregnancies

| | |
|---|---|
| Mean blood glucose (mg/dL) | 83.7 ± 18 |
| Fasting glucose (mg/dL) | 75 ± 12 |
| Preprandial glucose (mg/dL) | 78 ± 11 |
| Peak postprandial glucose value (mg/dL) | 110 ± 16 |
| Peak postprandial time (min) | 70 ± 13 |
| Mean blood glucose of 3-hour postprandial measurements (mg/dL) | 98 ± 12 |
| 1-hour postprandial glucose value (mg/dL) | 105 ± 13 |
| 2-hour postprandial glucose value (mg/dL) | 97 ± 11 |
| 3-hour postprandial glucose value (mg/dL) | 84 ± 14 |
| Mean blood glucose- night time (mg/dL) | 68 ± 10 |

nondiabetic controls [23]. No difference was obtained in postprandial glycemic profile between breakfast, lunch, or dinner. The question remains
whether the peak postprandial glucose or the time to return to preprandial
value will be a better reflection of quality of control. However, because all
the thresholds that are recommended currently (140 mg/dL at 1 hour and
120 mg/dL at 2 hours) are not related to preprandial values, it is reasonable
to speculate that the glucose value at the 90-minute intervals should be the
reflection of achievement of level of control. This idea is supported by the
finding in the authors' study that, in patients who have well-controlled diabetes mellitus, the peak glucose value was $103 \pm 26$ mg/dL; and in patients
whose diabetes mellitus was poorly controlled, the peak value was $164 \pm$
53 mg/dL.

Thus, it would be logical to combine both studies [23,24] and to suggest
that blood glucose determinations should be taken at 90 minutes post meal
with a desired glucose value of approximately 110 mg/dL. Nevertheless, the
authors recognize that future studies qualified by the frequency and timing
of testing are needed for evaluating the association between pregnancy outcome and these glycemic goals before advocating using these criteria for
routine management guidelines.

## Using continuous glucose monitoring for treatment assessment

Consensus exists that normoglycemia is desirable in the management of
diabetic pregnancies; however, the degree of deviation from normality characterized in daily glycemic profiles is poorly defined.

The wide range of glucose values obtained with the use of the CGM
provides the opportunity to identify both unrecognized hyperglycemia and
hypoglycemic events in comparison to self-monitoring blood glucose.

The authors used continuous glucose monitoring to assess the glycemic
profile in comparison to routine self-blood glucose monitoring in diabetic
pregnancies. The authors showed [25] that mean total time of undetected
hyperglycemia averaged 90 and 130 min/day for diet- and insulin-treated
GDM, respectively. Conversely, hypoglycemic events (defined as blood glucose less than 50 mg/day) were evaluated using continuous glucose monitoring [25,26]. The authors identified hypoglycemic events (most of them
asymptomatic) in approximately 60% of insulin-treated patients who had
GDM and in 28% of glyburide-treated patients. No hypoglycemic events
were identified in patients who had GDM treated by diet alone or in nondiabetic subjects. The mean recorded hypoglycemic episodes per day were
significantly higher in insulin-treated patients. The authors' data suggest
that asymptomatic hypoglycemic events are common during pharmacologic
treatment in gestational diabetic pregnancies. They speculate that this
finding may be explained by treatment modality rather than by the disease
pathophysiology itself. Clinical implications of these findings on pregnancy
outcome are still a matter of further study.

*Can continuous glucose monitoring be used for treatment adjustment?*

In a pilot study, the authors studied [27] eight women who had diabetes in pregnancy, of whom six were type 1, and two were GDM. Data derived from the CGM for 72 hours were assessed and treatment was adjusted on the basis of the findings. Two to 4 weeks later, the patients were re-evaluated with CGM. In the second period, a significant reduction in mean blood glucose, hypoglycemic events, and duration of undetected hyperglycemia was demonstrated. Recently, Kerssen and colleagues [28] reported that because there is a wide variability in the day-to-day glucose levels of pregnant women who have type 1 diabetes, the use of CGM raises a problem for adjustment of therapy. They concluded that fine-tuning of insulin regimens based on 3-day measurements with the CGM method is not advisable.

To respond to the previous subheading query, several conditions need to be met. A sample size should be large enough to provide data on pregnancy outcome; the study should include at least two groups, one using self-monitoring blood glucose, and the second, CGM and glucose testing must be performed throughout pregnancy because a 3-day testing cannot predict level of glycemia. These are the limitations of the current research using CMG. However, we need to be mindful that CGM is still an experimental measure and not a routine clinical tool. The frequency needed for CGM monitoring in diabetic pregnancy and its hypothetical advantage over self-monitoring blood glucose in enhancing pregnancy outcome still needs to be demonstrated.

## Subcutaneous continuous insulin infusion—insulin pump

*General considerations*

Insulin pumps were introduced in the late 1970s. There was initial excitement over this new technology, but within a few years their popularity weaned because their size, safety, and efficacy became a troublesome issue. Insulin pumps had resurgence in popularity after the Diabetes Control and Complications Trial (DCCT) results [29] were published. The new and modern pumps are smaller, more efficacious, easier to use, and safe. There are many commercially available insulin pumps manufactured by different companies that all operate similarly. The insulin pump contains an insulin-filled cartridge or a syringe connected to a catheter that is inserted into the subcutaneous tissue. The pump continuously delivers predetermined basal rates of insulin to meet nonprandial insulin requirements. The pump allows programming of different basal infusion rated and it also infuses a patient-control bolus to cover mealtime or snacktime insulin requirement.

*Glycemic control and adverse events in nonpregnancy*

In nonpregnant subjects, a meta-analysis performed on 12 randomized controlled trials of subcutaneous continuous insulin infusion (CSII) versus multiple injection regimens, whereby data were reliably extractable [30], showed a weighted mean difference in blood glucose concentration of 0.9 mmol/L (95% confidence interval 0.5–1.2) and a glycated hemoglobin difference of 0.5% (0.2–0.7) between CSII and optimized injection therapy, favoring CSII. The slightly but significantly better control on CSII was achieved with a 14% average reduction in daily insulin dose. In addition, CSII has been shown to decrease glycemic variability [31,32] and lower fasting glucose values [33,34].

*Potential disadvantages and side effects in using insulin pumps*

Importantly, studies have shown that pump therapy is associated with severe hypoglycemia. This notion was based from early case reports of episodes of hypoglycemic coma during CSII [35] and from the fact that the DCCT [29] found that the rate of severe hypoglycemia during CSII was approximately three times more frequent than during conventional injection therapy. Much of the DCCT-associated hypoglycemia may have been due to unfamiliarity with management of tight control because hypoglycemia rates halved during the course of the trial. Conversely, in a randomized crossover trial of CSII versus insulin injection therapy [36], it was demonstrated that the number of mild and moderate hypoglycemic episodes was reduced by nearly 60% by pump treatment. More recent reports have suggested that severe hypoglycemic events may be reduced as much as fourfold compared with multiple daily injections (MDI) of insulin [37,38] with no reduction in glycemic control. Severe hypoglycemic events have now become an accepted indication for CSII therapy.

A few early studies indicated a high rate of ketoacidosis with CSII [39,40]. But as patients and caregivers became more experienced with the technique, the frequency of ketoacidosis decreased [41]. Several remediable factors increased the likelihood of ketoacidosis during the first experiences with CSII, including physician inexperience (poor choice of infusion rates, poor instructions to patients, and so forth), the use of unbuffered insulin (which can cause cannula blockage), cannula dislodgment or leakage, and unsuitable patients (poorly compliant). There is no subcutaneous depot of long-acting insulin with CSII. If the flow of the regular short-acting insulin is interrupted, ketonuria and ketoacidosis can develop more rapidly and more frequently with CSII than with MDI [42].

The most common complication associated with CSII is infection at the infusion site [39]; moreover, this is the most common cause for discontinuation of CSII. Rarely, the infection may lead to cellulites and abscess formation.

A major disadvantage is the fact that the insulin pump and the supplies needed to begin therapy average approximately $5000. Moreover, the infusion set and catheters must be renewed regularly, which greatly contributes to the annually costs.

## The use of subcutaneous continuous insulin infusion in pregnancy complicated by diabetes

Most pregnancies complicated by diabetes are gestational in which diagnosis is established usually during the third trimester. This fact makes CSII treatment for GDM of modest relevance, if at all. Although major advances occurred in recent years in the treatment during pregnancy in women who have type 1 and 2 diabetes mellitus, still pregnancy is associated with an increased risk of congenital malformations, perinatal mortality, obstetric complications, and neonatal morbidity [43–49].

It is recognized that both CSII and MDI offer the advantage of frequent dose adjustment, which should lead to optimum blood sugar level attainment. It is less clear, due to the lack of any systematic meta-analysis or randomized studies of the evidence concerning the use of these different methods of administration during pregnancy, which method achieves the best outcome in terms of normalizing blood sugar level and reducing hypo/hyperglycemia to prevent associated complications for both mother and child.

Rosenn and colleagues [50] reported clinically significant hypoglycemia requiring assistance from another person in approximately 70% of type 1 pregnant patients. With the advantages of CSII in decreasing hypoglycemia and improving glycemic variability, it is logical to assume that CSII would be beneficial for pregnant women who have diabetes, especially during the first trimester.

Some studies suggest that CSII is superior to conventional therapy [51,52]; however these studies were limited by study sample and assessed only one aspect of pregnancy outcome (rate of congenital anomalies). Other studies have demonstrated comparable pregnancy outcome in CSII and MDI patients [53–55]. However, these studies were limited by different definitions for pre-GDM; only few evaluated level of glycemic control or firmly defined pregnancy outcome. A recent study has noted that women who initiate pump therapy during pregnancy are highly likely to continue with the pump after they deliver. They maintain better glucose control than do patients remaining on multiple insulin injections [56,57]. Lapolla and colleagues [58] compared metabolic control and maternal outcome in CSII and MDI type 1 patients during pregnancy. No differences were observed between the two groups in pregnancy outcome and especially in malformation rate.

It is understandable that patient's satisfaction and lifestyle flexibility is increased under CSII treatment in comparison to MDI treatment. CSII allows the patients to modify insulin availability hour by hour and to avoid multiple injections during the day. This increased flexibility, especially during pregnancy may be fueling the upsurge in patient demand for CSII more than any other factor. Nevertheless, to establish clear benefit of CSII (other than improvement in lifestyle) as regarding pregnancy outcome, a large prospective randomized study is needed.

## The future: a closed-loop system (an artificial pancreas)

"Closed loop" system means one system that monitors for glucose levels and accordingly supplies insulin. The ideal closed-loop system, or "artificial pancreas," should contain three key elements: (1) a safe-delivery device that stores and releases insulin reliably and accurately; (2) an accurate, biocompatible glucose-sensing unit capable of frequent or continuous sampling; and (3) a control system that modulates delivery of insulin, glucose, and maybe glucagon or amylin, according to blood glucose levels. Additionally, the miniature computer system in an artificial pancreas must be able to sample, filter, and interpret the glucose sensor data, to compare the reading with allowable norms, and to accurately control insulin to maintain normoglycemia. This process must operate correctly all the time, to avoid errors leading to severe hypo- or hyperglycemia.

Efforts to connect the CSII system with a real-time glucose sensor have already been reported in animal models and even some human trials [57]. Operating together, the glucose sensors and insulin pumps should, in effect, serve as an artificial pancreas, mimicking the role of the pancreatic beta cells and freeing the patient from the need for constant daily care of his/her food intake, physical activities, and insulin doses. Wireless transmission between implantable pump and glucose sensor has been accomplished as well. The Paradigm® 522/722 sensor-augmented insulin pump system (Medtronic MiniMed) is a fully external system designed to use a subcutaneous glucose sensor, which is easily inserted under the skin, to continuously record blood sugar readings for up to 3 days. The system's transmitter sends continuous glucose readings by way of radio frequency to the pump, which displays real-time glucose readings every 5 minutes, in addition to trend graphs and hypoglycemia and hyperglycemia alerts to the patient to make immediate corrective adjustments by way of the pump. So far, however, the glucose sensor and the insulin pump are unable to "talk" to each other, so the patients' input and decision-making are still necessary. This technology was not yet studied in pregnancy. Unfortunately, the accuracy of the current continuous glucose sensors and algorithms is not yet sufficient to permit the loop to be closed. In the meantime, patients can enjoy the technologic innovations that are already available. The new and improved "smart" insulin pumps and the next generation of "real-time" continuous glucose sensors can still serve as helpful tools. It may be that implantation of this technology into diabetes in pregnancy will be associated with perinatal outcome similar to nondiabetic subjects.

## References

[1] Suhonen L, Hiilesmaa V, Teramo K. Glycemic control during early pregnancy and fetal malformations in women with type 1 diabetes mellitus. Diabetologia 2000;43:79–82.
[2] Lauenborg J, Mathiesen E, Ovesen P, et al. Audit on stillbirths in women with pregestational type 1 diabetes. Diabetes Care 2003;26(5):1385–8.

[3] Platt MJ, Stanisstreet M, Casson IF, et al. St. Vincent's declaration 10 years on: outcomes of diabetic pregnancies. Diabet Med 2002;19:216–20.
[4] Ostlund I, Hanson U, Bjorklund A, et al. Maternal and fetal outcomes if gestational impaired glucose tolerance is not treated. Diabetes Care 2003;26(7):2107–11.
[5] Widness JA, Schwartz HC, Kahn CB, et al. Glycohemoglobin in diabetic pregnancy: a sequential study. Am J Obstet Gynecol 1980;136:1024–9.
[6] Phelps RL, Honig GR, Green D, et al. Biphasic changes in hemoglobin A1c concentrations during normal human pregnancy. Am J Obstet Gynecol 1983;147:651–3.
[7] Hall PM, Cook JGH, Sheldon J, et al. Glycosylated hemoglobins and glycosylated plasma proteins in the diagnosis of diabetes mellitus and impaired glucose tolerance. Diabetes Care 1984;7:147–50.
[8] Langer O, Mazze R. The relationship between glycosylated haemoglobin and verified self-monitored blood glucose among pregnant and non-pregnant women with diabetes. Practical Diabetes 1987;4(1):32–3.
[9] Brustman L, Langer O, Engel S, et al. Verified self-monitored blood glucose data versus glycosylated hemoglobin and glycosylated serum protein as a means of predicting short-and long-term metabolic control in gestational diabetes. Am J Obstet Gynecol 1987;157(3):699–703.
[10] Cocilovo G, Guerra S, Colla F, et al. Glycosylated hemoglobin (HbA1) assay as a test for detection and surveillance of gestational diabetes. A reappraisal. Diabete Metab 1987;13(4):426–30.
[11] Loke DF, Chua S, Kek LP, et al. Glycosylated hemoglobins in pregnant women with normal and abnormal glucose tolerance. Gynecol Obstet Invest 1994;37(1):25–9.
[12] Wyse LJ, Jones M, Mandel F. Relationship of glycosylated hemoglobin, fetal macrosomia, and birthweight macrosomia. Am J Perinatol 1994;11(4):260–2.
[13] Weissmann-Brenner A, O'Reilly-Green C, Ferber A, et al. Does the availability of maternal HbA1c results improve the accuracy of sonographic diagnosis of macrosomia? Ultrasound Obstet Gynecol 2004;23(5):466–71.
[14] Langer O, Rodriguez DA, Xenakis EMJ, et al. Intensified versus conventional management of gestational diabetes. Am J Obstet Gynecol 1994;170(4):1036–47.
[15] Mastrototaro J. The MiniMed continuous glucose monitoring system (CGMS). J Pediatr Endocrinol Metab 1999;12(Suppl 3):751–8.
[16] Garg SK, Potts RO, Ackerman NR, et al. Correlation of finger stick blood glucose measurements with Glucowatch Biographer glucose results in young subjects with type 1 diabetes. Diabetes Care 1999;22:1708–14.
[17] Rebrin K, Steil GM, van Antwerp WP, et al. Subcutaneous glucose predicts plasma glucose independent of insulin: implications for continuous monitoring. Am J Physiol 1999;277:E561–71.
[18] Gerritsen M, Jansen JA, Lutterman JA. Performance of subcutaneously implanted glucose sensors for continuous monitoring. Neth J Med 1999;54:167–79.
[19] Gillmer MD, Beard RW, Brooke FM, et al. Carbohydrate metabolism in pregnancy. Part I. Diurnal plasma glucose profile in normal and diabetic women. Br Med J 1975;3(5980):399–402.
[20] Cousins L, Rigg L, Hollingsworth D, et al. The 24-hour excursion and diurnal rhythm of glucose, insulin, and C-peptide in normal pregnancy. Am J Obstet Gynecol 1980;136(4):483–8.
[21] Phelps RL, Metzger BE, Freinkel N. Carbohydrate metabolism in pregnancy. XVII. Diurnal profiles of plasma glucose, insulin, free fatty acids, triglycerides, cholesterol, and individual amino acids in late normal pregnancy. Am J Obstet Gynecol 1981;140(7):730–6.
[22] Parretti E, Mecacci F, Papini M, et al. Third-trimester maternal glucose levels from diurnal profiles in nondiabetic pregnancies: correlation with sonographic parameters of fetal growth. Diabetes Care 2001;24(8):1319–23.
[23] Yogev Y, Ben-Haroush A, Chen R, et al. Diurnal glycemic profile in obese and normal weight non-diabetic pregnant women. Am J Obstet Gynecol 2004;191(3):949–53.

[24] Ben-Haroush A, Yogev Y, Chen R, et al. The postprandial glucose profile in the diabetic pregnancy. Am J Obstet Gynecol 2004;191(2):576–81.

[25] Chen R, Yogev Y, Ben-Haroush A, et al. Continuous glucose monitoring for the evaluation and improved control of gestational diabetes mellitus. J Matern Fetal Neonatal Med 2003; 14(4):256–60.

[26] Yogev Y, Ben-Haroush A, Chen R, et al. Undiagnosed asymptomatic hypoglycemia: diet, insulin, and glyburide for gestational diabetic pregnancy. Obstet Gynecol 2004;104(1): 88–93.

[27] Yogev Y, Ben-Haroush A, Chen R, et al. Continuous glucose monitoring for treatment adjustment in diabetic pregnancies—a pilot study. Diabet Med 2003;20(7):558–62.

[28] Kerssen A, de Valk HW, Visser GH. Day-to-day glucose variability during pregnancy in women with type 1 diabetes mellitus: glucose profiles measured with the continuous glucose monitoring system. BJOG 2004;111(9):919–24.

[29] The diabetes control and complications trial research group. The effect of intensive treatment of diabetes on the development and progression of long-term complications in insulin-dependent diabetes mellitus. The Diabetes Control and Complications Trial Research Group. N Engl J Med 1993;329:977–86.

[30] Pickup J, Mattock M, Kerry S. Glycemic control with continuous subcutaneous insulin infusion compared with intensive insulin injections in patients with type 1 diabetes: meta-analysis of randomized controlled trials. BMJ 2002;324(7339):705.

[31] Bischof F, Meyerhoff C, Pfeiffer EF. Quality control of intensified insulin therapy: HbA1 versus blood glucose. Horm Metab Res 1994;26(12):574–8.

[32] Lauritzen T, Pramming S, Deckert T, et al. Pharmacokinetics of continuous subcutaneous insulin infusion. Diabetologia 1983;24(5):326–9.

[33] Koivisto VA, Yki-Jarvinen H, Helve E, et al. Pathogenesis and prevention of the dawn phenomenon in diabetic patients treated with CSII. Diabetes 1986;35(1):78–82.

[34] Schiffrin A, Belmonte MM. Comparison between continuous subcutaneous insulin infusion and multiple injections of insulin. A one-year prospective study. Diabetes 1982;31(3):255–64.

[35] Locke DR, Rigg LA. Hypoglycemic coma associated with subcutaneous insulin infusion by portable pump. Diabetes Care 1981;4:389–91.

[36] Ng Tang Fui S, Pickup JC, Bending JJ, et al. Hypoglycemia and counterregulation in insulin-dependent diabetic patients: a comparison of continuous subcutaneous insulin infusion and conventional insulin therapy. Diabetes Care 1986;9:221–7.

[37] Bode BW, Steed RD, Davidson PC. Reduction in severe hypoglycemia with long-term continuous subcutaneous insulin infusion in type I diabetes. Diabetes Care 1996;19(4):324–7.

[38] Haardt MJ, Berne C, Dorange C, et al. Efficacy and indications of CSII revisited: the Hotel-Dieu cohort. Diabet Med 1997;14(5):407–8.

[39] Mecklenburg RS, Benson EA, Benson JW, et al. Acute complications associated with insulin infusion pump therapy. Report of experience with 161 patients. JAMA 1984;252(23):3265–9.

[40] Knight G, Jennings AM, Boulton AJM, et al. Severe hyperglycaemia and ketoacidosis during routine treatment with an insulin pump. BMJ 1985;291:371–2.

[41] Bending JJ, Pickup JC, Keen H. Frequency of diabetic ketoacidosis and hypoglycemic coma during treatment with continuous subcutaneous insulin infusion. Am J Med 1985;79:685–91.

[42] Pickup JC, Viberti GC, Bilous RW, et al. Safety of continuous subcutaneous insulin infusion: metabolic deterioration and glycaemic autoregulation after deliberate cessation of infusion. Diabetologia 1992;22:175–9.

[43] Barfield W, Martin J, Hoyert D. Racial/ethnic trends in fetal mortality in United States, 1990–2000. MMWR Morb Mortal Wkly Rep 2004;53:529–32.

[44] Hawthorne G, Robson S, Ryall EA, et al. Prospective population based survey of outcome of pregnancy in diabetic women: results of the northern diabetic pregnancy audit, 1994. BMJ 1997;315:279–81.

[45] Casson IF, Clarke CA, Howard CV, et al. Outcomes of pregnancy in insulin dependent diabetic women: results of a five year population cohort study. BMJ 1997;315:275–8.

[46] Vaarasmaki M, Gissler M, Ritvanen A, et al. Congenital anomalies and first year life surveillance in type 1 diabetic births. Diabet Med 2002;19:589–93.

[47] Diabetes and pregnancy group, France. French multicentric survey of outcome of pregnancy in women with pregestational diabetes. Diabetes Care 2003;26:2990–3.

[48] Evers IM, de Valk HW, Visser GH. Risk of complications of pregnancy in women with type 1 diabetes: nationwide prospective study in the Netherlands. BMJ 2004;328:915–20.

[49] Penney GC, Mair G, Pearson DW, Scottish Diabetes in Pregnancy Group. Outcomes of pregnancies in women with type 1 diabetes in Scotland: a national population-based study. BJOG 2003;110(3):315–8.

[50] Rosenn BM, Miodovnik M, Holcberg G, et al. Hypoglycemia: the price of intensive insulin therapy for pregnant women with insulin-dependent diabetes mellitus. Obstet Gynecol 1995; 85(3):417–22.

[51] Kitzmiller JL, Gavin LA, Gin GD, et al. Preconception care of diabetes. Glycemic control prevents congenital anomalies. JAMA 1991;265(6):731–6.

[52] Jensen BM, Kuhl C, Molsted-Pedersen L, et al. Preconceptional treatment with insulin infusion pumps in insulin-dependent diabetic women with particular reference to prevention of congenital malformations. Acta Endocrinol Suppl (Copenh) 1986;277:81–5.

[53] Potter JM, Reckless JP, Cullen DR. The effect of continuous subcutaneous insulin infusion and conventional insulin regimes on 24-hour variations of blood glucose and intermediary metabolites in the third trimester of diabetic pregnancy. Diabetologia 1981;21(6):534–9.

[54] Burkart W, Hanker JP, Schneider HP. Complications and fetal outcome in diabetic pregnancy. Intensified conventional versus insulin pump therapy. Gynecol Obstet Invest 1988;26(2):104–12.

[55] Carta Q, Meriggi E, Trossarelli GF, et al. Continuous subcutaneous insulin infusion versus intensive conventional insulin therapy in type I and type II diabetic pregnancy. Diabete Metab 1986;12(3):121–9.

[56] Gabbe SG, Holing E, Temple P, et al. Benefits, risks, costs, and patient satisfaction associated with insulin pump therapy for the pregnancy complicated by type 1 diabetes mellitus. Am J Obstet Gynecol 2000;182:1283–91.

[57] Renard E, Shah R, Miller M, et al. Sustained safety and accuracy of central IV glucose sensors connected to implanted insulin pumps and short-term closed-loop trials in diabetic patients. Diabetes 2003;52(Suppl 2):155.

[58] Lapolla A, Dalfra MG, Masin M, et al. Analysis of outcome of pregnancy in type 1 diabetics treated with insulin pump or conventional insulin therapy. Acta Diabetol 2003;40(3):143–9.

ELSEVIER
SAUNDERS

Obstet Gynecol Clin N Am
34 (2007) 255–274

OBSTETRICS AND
GYNECOLOGY
CLINICS
OF NORTH AMERICA

# Oral Anti-Hyperglycemic Agents for the Management of Gestational Diabetes Mellitus

## Oded Langer, MD, PhD

*Department of Obstetrics and Gynecology, St. Luke's-Roosevelt Hospital Center,
Women's Health Service, University Hospital of Columbia University,
1000 10th Avenue, 10 C-01, New York, NY 10019, USA*

The purpose of this review is to provide a brief overview for understanding the management guidelines of gestational diabetes. The rationale for the use of oral antidiabetic drugs is provided based on validation by appropriately conducted research trials [1]. Concerns over teratogenicity due to possible placental transfer, neonatal and maternal outcome, and basic pharmacologic benefits are addressed.

Gestational diabetes mellitus (GDM) is defined as carbohydrate intolerance first diagnosed during pregnancy. This definition, however, is problematic because several million type 2 diabetic women remain undiagnosed until the disease is first recognized during pregnancy. These women, in all likelihood, are classified as GDM. Thus, GDM actually represents a mix of women who have had abnormal tolerance test results in pregnancy and undiagnosed type 2 diabetes. The prevalence of GDM varies in direct proportion to the prevalence of type 2 diabetes in a given population, ethnic group, or geographic area. Therefore, different studies may report varying rates of population prevalence, complications, and so forth. In the United States, the prevalence rate ranges from 1% to 14% [1].

In addition to the undiagnosed type 2 diabetic women that are masked in the GDM population, couldn't GDM be "early" type 2 diabetes and thus represent the same disease with a different name? It is the similarities between type 2 and gestational diabetes in risk factors and metabolic and endocrine abnormalities that provide the rationale for proposing that they are the same disease. Type 2 diabetes and GDM are heterogeneous disorders whose pathophysiology is characterized by peripheral insulin resistance,

---

*E-mail address:* odlanger@chpnet.org

0889-8545/07/$ - see front matter © 2007 Elsevier Inc. All rights reserved.
doi:10.1016/j.ogc.2007.03.004

impaired regulation of hepatic glucose production, and declining β-cell function. The primary events are deficits in insulin secretion, followed by peripheral insulin resistance. Glucose intolerance follows β-cell dysfunction (impairment in the first phase of insulin secretion). In the second phase, the release of newly synthesized insulin is impaired. When tight glycemic control is achieved, it can reverse the effects of glucose toxicity that produce the intrapancreatic (desensitization of β-cells) or extrapancreatic effect [2,3].

It has become axiomatic that the goal of treatment of pregnant and nonpregnant diabetic patients is to optimize the glycemic profile. This is customarily performed in the pregnant diabetic with the trial of diet therapy and the addition of pharmacologic therapy (insulin or oral antidiabetic drugs such as glyburide) when glycemic control cannot be achieved by diet alone [4]. Therefore, several authors selected to use achievement of blood glucose control as the primary outcome variable when comparing drugs designed to reduce levels of glycemia [5,6].

Insulin and oral antidiabetic agents were designed to reduce the level of glycemia; this parallels the use of drugs designed to reduce hypertension or cholesterol. These drugs have been accepted as valid measures for achieving control over specific diseases. If and when these drugs achieve the task for which they were designed, then secondary outcomes are used to determine whether they can prevent heart attack, stroke, or, as in the case of gestational diabetes, adverse maternal and fetal outcomes.

### The role of pharmacology in the treatment of gestational diabetes mellitus

Several questions need to be addressed when pharmacologic therapy is under consideration. *Who* is the appropriate recipient? *How long* should a patient be treated solely with diet before pharmacologic treatment is initiated? *When* should a patient be evaluated for glycemic profile?

There are two thresholds for the initiation of pharmacologic therapy. The traditional threshold requires fasting plasma glucose greater than or equal to 105 mg/dL, whereas the more intensified approach uses fasting plasma glucose greater than or equal to 95 mg/dL in conjunction with post meal levels greater than or equal to 120 mg/dL for 2 hours or 140 mg/dL for 1 hour. Based on these criteria, for a given population, approximately 30% to 50% of women who have GDM will require pharmacologic therapy when diet alone fails to reduce glycemic levels [4,7]. However, it has recently been suggested that to obtain improved perinatal outcome in obese women who have GDM, they will need to be treated with pharmacologic (insulin) even in the presence of good glycemic control with diet alone [8]. Thus, the rate of patients who have GDM who require pharmacologic therapy can be even higher than previously suggested.

Although there is paucity of information regarding the length of time that diet should be maintained before initiation of pharmacologic therapy, we need to note that the time from diagnosis to delivery in GDM is short. Most patients who have GDM are diagnosed between 28 and 32 weeks and deliver between 37 and 39 weeks of gestation. The delay in pharmacologic therapy initiation with its potential to achieve the established levels of glycemic control will result in irreversible adverse outcome (macrosomia, metabolic complications, and so forth).

For patients who have a threshold fasting plasma of less than 95 mg/dL and, therefore, qualified for the trial of diet therapy, a 2-week diet-alone period will identify most patients who successfully achieved the desired level of glycemic control [9]. Therefore, obese GDM (body mass index > 29) and patients who have fasting plasma greater than 95 mg/dL or those who have fasting plasma glucose less than 95 mg/dL who failed to achieve the desired level of glycemic control within 2 weeks, required pharmacologic therapy. Still, for every valid recommendation, there is a valid exception; in these cases, the practitioner's clinical wisdom supercedes the recommendation. For example, in a case whereby GDM is diagnosed after 28 to 30 weeks of gestation and there is less time to influence the desired level of control, the care provider needs to be more liberal in the early initiation of pharmacologic therapy. In contrast, there will be more flexibility when GDM is diagnosed during the second trimester, when the growth stimulation to the fetus is not yet prominent.

## Oral antidiabetic drugs in gestational diabetes mellitus treatment

The rationale for the use of antidiabetic agents is motivated by three main factors:

1. GDM and patients who have impaired glucose tolerance have a mild hyperglycemia in comparison to type 2 diabetic individuals. Because oral antidiabetic agents can decrease the glycemic profile in type 2 diabetes, it is reasonable to speculate that they will be even more effective in the treatment of GDM.
2. There is a similarity in the pathogenesis of type 2 diabetes and GDM. In addition to the insulin secretion and resistance abnormalities found in both conditions, there is a loss of the first-phase insulin secretion with a striking lag time between the postprandial rise in glucose and the presence of significant insulin at the peripheral sites. This will result in an early increase in postprandial glucose values. Because second-generation sulfonylurea agents are rapid in onset and have short duration of action, it makes them ideal agents to treat very early stages of type 2 and possibly GDM patients.
3. The United Kingdom Prospective Diabetes Study [10] of type 2 diabetes supported the efficacy of these drugs and in particular the use of glyburide.

Regardless of the success of the intensified treatment model [7], a less invasive, more patient-friendly alternative that enhances patient compliance while achieving similar perinatal outcome is a welcome replacement. Oral antidiabetic agents are convenient to use, less invasive than insulin, and less expensive. Therefore, they can become the drug of choice when dietary modifications fail to reduce hyperglycemia. Oral antidiabetic agents are used in the United States especially to provide patients who have type 2 diabetes support in maintaining the tight glucose control that lowers their risk for microvascular complications (Table 1).

Both the United Kingdom Prospective Diabetes Study (UKPDS) [10] and the DCCT [11] strongly support the use of intensive therapy in patients who

Table 1
Studies reporting successful treatment of oral antidiabetic agents in pregnancy

| Study | Study design | Type of diabetes | No. of patient | | Achievement of good control |
|---|---|---|---|---|---|
| | | | Glyburide | Regular insulin | |
| Langer, 2000 [6] | RCT | GDM | 201 | 203 | 82% and 88% |
| Lim, 1997 [53] | Prosp, observ | GDM | 33 | 21 | No significant difference |
| Conway, 2004 [54] | Prosp, observ | GDM | 75 | — | 84% |
| Kremer, 2004 [55] | Prosp, observ | GDM | 73 | — | 81% |
| Chmait, 2004 [56] | Prosp, observ | GDM | 69 | — | 82% |
| Gilson, 2002 [57] | Prosp, observ | GDM | 22 | 22 | 82% |
| Fines, 2003 [58] | Retro (case control) | GDM | 40 | 44 | NA |
| Velazques, 2003 [59] | Case Series | GDM | 31 | 7 | Glyburide 82% |
| Pendsey, 2002 [60] | RCT | Type 2 | — | 23 | Improved level of glycemic control |
| Coetzee, 1979 [21] | Prosp, observ | GDM & Type 2 | | GDM: 81.4% | |
| Hellmuth, 2000 [52] | Prosp, observ | GDM | Sulfonylurea:68 | 42 | Type 2 diabetes 46.2% |
| Notelowitz, 1971 [18] | RCT | GDM & Type 2 | Tolbutamide chlorpropamin: 2x 52 | 52 | Using oral hypoglycemic: 80% |
| Yogev, 2004 [65] | Prosp | GDM | 25 | 30 | Mean blood glucose similar in all groups |
| Moore, 2005 | RCT | GDM | Metformin: 32 | 31 | Blood glucose similar |
| Jacobson, 2005 [61] | Retro | GDM | 236 | 316 | Blood glucose similar |

*Abbreviations:* Observ, observational; Props, prospective; RCT, randomized control trial; Retro, retrospective.

have type 1 and type 2 diabetes to achieve and maintain near-normal HbA1c levels and to prevent diabetic complications. These pivotal studies, including the author's practice's large prospective study of over 2000 patients who have GDM [7], challenge health care professionals to implement standards for improved glycemic control with the intent of decreasing the complications of the disease.

The UKPDS, the largest prospective study evaluating the impact of oral antidiabetic agents on the outcome of type 2 diabetes, demonstrated that in 70% of the patients, a desirable level of glucose control was achieved with the use of sulfonylurea-glyburide. The most favorable effect was obtained within the first 5 years of the disease (70% of the patients treated with glyburide achieved the desired goal). In years 3, 6, and 9, the desired goals were achieved by fewer than 55%, 40%, and 30% of patients, respectively, using a single agent (insulin, sulfonylurea, or metformin). With greater deterioration in β-cell function, multiple therapies will eventually be needed in most patients to achieve glycemic target levels [10].

The study also demonstrated a 25% reduction of risk, primarily attributed to microvascular complications and a trend toward fewer macrovascular complications after intensive therapy versus conventional therapy. Improved glycemic control rather than a specific therapy was the primary factor responsible for the reduced risk of complications, because all treatments (eg, insulin, glyburide, metformin) had similar risk reduction. In comparison to the UKPDS success rate in achieving glycemic control in type 2 diabetes with the use of glyburide, women who have GDM who are characterized by a milder glycemic profile should have an equal or greater success in achieving glycemic control with the use of antidiabetic agents.

## Oral hypoglycemic agents

In Europe and in South Africa, first-generation sulphonylureas, glyburide and metformin, have been used for years [12–22]. The fierce resistance against the use of these agents in pregnancy stems from the lack of data from well-designed studies (ie, retrospective studies with small sample sizes). In general, outcome-based research is not always available. As a result, this was the driving force behind the creation of the US Preventive Services Task Force criterion for the review and evaluation of studies. The highest level of research study is evidence obtained from at least one properly designed randomized controlled trial, followed by controlled trials without randomization and cohort or case-controlled analytic studies. The lowest level of quality is the opinions of respected authorities based on clinical experience, descriptive studies, or reports of expert committees [1].

In the United States, up until the year 2000, the use of oral antidiabetic drugs (hypoglycemic or antihyperglycemic) was contraindicated [23–25]. Therefore, they have played a limited role in the management of GDM in the United States. The main objection to their use in pregnancy is the risk for the development of congenital anomalies, fetal compromise, and fetal hypoglycemic episodes through direct stimulation of the fetal pancreas [26–28]. The historic ban on the use of oral hypoglycemic agents in pregnancy have been based on scant evidence of case reports [26–28] and one study in particular on fetal anomalies in 50 poorly controlled diabetic women before pregnancy [29] begging the question: Is it the drug or is it the glucose?

Therefore, up until recently, the American College of Obstetrics and Gynecologists and the American Diabetes Association did not recommend the use of oral hypoglycemic agents [24,25]. It is only recently in the United States that consideration of the use of oral hypoglycemic agents in pregnancy has become debatable and then accepted practice by scientific forums (North American Diabetes in Pregnancy Study Group and the 5th International Workshop on Gestational Diabetes).

The concerns regarding the use of oral hypoglycemic agents in the treatment of GDM were recently studied in a systematic format with adequate sample size and randomized design [6]. This study demonstrated that glyburide is comparable to insulin in achieving maternal levels of glycemia that result in a perinatal outcome similar to that in the general population [6].

## Sulfonylureas

Sulfonylureas have been used to treat type 2 diabetes for many decades and require functional pancreatic β-cell for their hypoglycemic effect. They bind to specific receptors (SUR1: sulphonylureas, repaglinide, nateglinide) on β-cell plasma membrane, resulting in closure of potassium adenosine triphosphate channels. As a result, calcium channels open, leading to an increase in cytoplasmic calcium that stimulates insulin release. The primary effect of these drugs is to enhance insulin secretion [30,31]. Enhanced insulin secretion suppresses the production of hepatic glucose, the main contributor to fasting hyperglycemia. It diminishes glucose toxicity and improves insulin secretion after meals, thus reducing postprandial hyperglycemia. Studies have demonstrated [32–34] that these drugs can also enhance peripheral tissue sensitivity to insulin. The peak plasma level of glyburide when given as a single agent occurs within 4 hours. Food does not affect the absorption of the drug. Glyburide is extensively metabolized in the liver, and its metabolites are extracted in bile and urine to equal extent. The elimination half-life of glyburide is approximately 10 hours. Glibenclamide is synonymous with glyburide in Europe. The main side effect of glyburide is hypoglycemia that may occur in 11% to 38% of nonpregnant patients who have type 2 diabetes. The hypoglycemic symptoms are dose-related; the risk of a hypoglycemic episode is greater for the older patient.

The ideal patient for this therapy is either of normal weight or obese, has been hyperglycemic for less than 5 years and is willing to follow a dietary program. β-cell exhaustion and insulin resistance are characteristic features of type 2 diabetes and GDM. Moreover, the phenotypic features of these complications are similar (ie, both are obese and asymptomatic) (at least in the early stages of the disease), with similar prevalence in the same ethnic group. Therefore, the use of a sulfonylurea agent could be beneficial in the prevention of GDM complications.

The author's practice demonstrated [35–37] that second-generation oral hypoglycemic agents, especially glyburide, do not significantly cross the diabetic or nondiabetic placenta. Fetal concentrations reached no more than 1% to 2% of maternal concentrations. The author's practice used a recirculating single-cotyledon placenta model in vitro to characterize the maternal-to-fetal term placentas perfused immediately following delivery. The author's practice further compared various sulfonylureas and found that tolbutamide diffused across the placenta most freely, followed by chlorpropamide, then glipizide, with glyburide crossing the least. Finally, in 2000, the author's practice conducted a randomized controlled trial comparing insulin and glyburide in the management of gestational diabetes [6]. The trial did not detect a measurable glyburide level in umbilical cord blood, despite the mothers having therapeutic concentrations of glyburide in their blood. To date, no study has measured fetal concentration of glyburide. The author's findings that glyburide did not cross the placenta were confirmed by several research groups. They further contributed to the explanation of why glyburide does not cross the placenta despite the fact that its molecular weight is less than 500. One explanation may be the high protein-binding capacity, 99.8% [38]. A potential problem is that albumin levels decrease physiologically, and thus there is increased transfer of glyburide. However, when this hypothesis was tested, it was shown that decreased albumin concentration associated with pregnancy is unlikely to affect the deposition of glyburide [39]. In addition, it was demonstrated in perfusion studies that glyburide is actively efflux by a transporter other than P-glycoprotein. Alternatively, it is possible that a smaller portion of glyburide is carried by P-glycoprotein, but most of the fetal load is pumped to the mother by an unidentified placental transport system [40]. The elimination of the threat of glyburide crossing the placenta and the adverse affects to the fetus (malformations and hypoglycemia) enhances the potential for the use of glyburide as a vigorous alternative pharmacologic agent in the management of patients who have GDM [6,41–45].

Glyburide can be expected to reduce fasting plasma glucose by 2 to 4 mmol/L accompanied by a decrease in HbA1c of 1% to 2% (a decrease of 1% = 20–30 mg glucose) [45–47]. Furthermore, its efficacy is maximized within the first 5 years of diagnosis. A continuous gradual loss of β-cell function is to be expected in most type 2 diabetic patients. This will require increased pharmacologic doses with longer disease duration. It is *not* reasonable to assume that within the 8- to 12-week window of GDM therapy with glyburide or any other oral antidiabetic agents, that the drug will either contribute to an escalation or deterioration of pancreatic function. In fact, if this was the case, no oral therapy with sulphonylureas or sulphony-lurea-like drugs could be used in the treatment of type 2 diabetes. Obviously, this is not the case. GDM patients who are characterized by mild hypergly-cemia are excellent candidates for therapy with glyburide or other oral antidiabetic drugs (metformin, α-gludosidase inhibitors, and thiazolidine-diones) as long as they are not transferred across the placenta. The potential ability of these agents to decrease levels of glycemia will facilitate achieving the targeted levels of glycemia required in pregnancy, which are much lower than those for the nonpregnant state [48–50].

The results of the placental transport studies and the mild hyperglycemia in most pregnant women who have GDM led the author to hypothesize that glyburide could be an alternative to insulin therapy. The author's practice enrolled 404 women who had GDM into a study. The blood glucose profile characteristics before initiation of therapy were comparable for the glybur-ide and the insulin-treated groups (114 ± 9 mg/dL versus 116 ± 22 mg/dL, respectively). During the treatment period, mean glucose values were similar (105 ± 16 versus 116 ± 22 mg/dL) as were fasting, preprandial and post-prandial values, and glycohemoglobin values. Eight glyburide-treated women (4%) who failed to achieve the desired level of control were trans-ferred to the insulin-therapy group. Eighty-two percent of the glyburide pa-tients and 80% of the insulin-treated women achieved the targeted levels of glycemic control. This finding was reconfirmed by several studies that dem-onstrated the efficacy of treatment with glyburide in obtaining targeted goals (Table 1) [51–61].

In another study, the author's practice stratified the glyburide patients by level of disease severity (using categories of fasting plasma glucose). They found an inverse relation between disease severity and level of glycemia result-ing in approximately 40% in the high fasting category achieving targeted levels of glycemic control. This was true for glyburide and insulin-treated pa-tients at each level of severity. Of note, the success rate in the high-severity cat-egory is similar to that reported in the nonpregnant type 2 diabetics [62–64].

Sulphonylureas can cause hypoglycemia because insulin release is initi-ated even when glucose concentration is below the normal threshold for glu-cose-stimulated insulin release (approximately 5 mmol/L or 90 mg/dL). Therefore, there was concern over the possibility of an increased rate of hypoglycemia with glyburide-treated patients. It should be understood that any therapy used in the treatment of diabetic patients in pregnancy (diet, insulin, oral antidiabetic agents) would be associated with a certain rate of hypoglycemic episodes. Furthermore, pregnancy by itself is prone to hypo-glycemia due to the phenomenon of accelerated starvation. Any attempt to evaluate hypoglycemic episodes needs to differentiate between patient-reported clinical episodes confirmed by glucose testing and accidentally found hypoglycemic glucose values on self-monitoring blood glucose results. The current self-monitoring technique from noninvasive to continuous blood glucose monitoring are all prone to testing errors and limited by the level of hypoglycemic values that they can measure.

The author's practice found, in a randomized study measuring blood glucose throughout the disease (GDM) period, a significant decrease in hypoglycemic episodes in the glyburide group in comparison to the insulin-treated patients [6]. In another study, using continuous blood glucose monitoring for 3 days, they reconfirmed their original findings; however, the testing time was limited. Their findings that hypoglycemia does not increase with the use of glyburide therapy in GDM was confirmed in another study [65].

Analysis of outcome variables when comparing glyburide and the insulin-treated groups demonstrated similar rates for pre-eclampsia (6% versus 6%) and Cesarean section (23% versus 24%). The rate of large for gestational age neonates was 12% versus 13%, macrosomia 7% versus 4%, and hypoglycemia 9% versus 6%. No significant differences were found in any of the primary or secondary outcome values; moreover, there was no identifiable trend that might suggest that an increased sample size could demonstrate a difference between the groups. The 95% confidence interval for the difference of the mean was found to be small and narrow. This result suggests a small likelihood of beta errors in this study. Again, several studies reconfirmed the author's findings that glyburide can help achieve the same perinatal outcome as insulin.

## Biguanides

Metformin is an insulin sensitizer that reduces insulin resistance and basal plasma insulin levels; therefore, it affects the glycemic profile. Metformin has various metabolic effects: it suppresses hepatic glucose output; increases insulin-mediated glucose use; decreases fatty acid oxidation; increases splanchnic glucose turnover; improves lipid profile by decreasing triglyceridemia, fatty acids, and low density lipoprotein (LDL) cholesterol while slightly increasing high density lipoprotein (HDL) cholesterol and decreasing intestinal absorption of glucose and use. In addition, it stabilizes or facilitates weight reduction. Metformin does not stimulate insulin secretion, and, therefore, does not cause hypoglycemia in either diabetic or control subjects. Metformin does not stimulate the fetal pancreas to oversecrete insulin.

Metformin is a second-generation biguanide introduced in the United States after the withdrawal of phenformin. Lactic acidosis is infrequent (0.03 cases/1000 patient-years), one-tenth that of the parent drug. The risk of lactic acidosis increases with the degree of renal dysfunction and patient age. Its peak plasma level given as a single agent occurs within 4 hours. The extent of absorption is reduced in the presence of food, although it should be administered with meals to minimize gastrointestinal intolerance. In contrast to glyburide, which is extensively metabolized in the liver, metformin is not metabolized and is eliminated unchanged in the urine. Peak plasma concentrations are short-lived; in patients who have normal renal function, the plasma half-life (t1/2) for metformin is 2 to 5 hours with almost 90% of an absorbed dosage eliminated within 12 hours [66,67]. Renal clearance of metformin occurs more often by tubular secretion than glomerular filtration with minimal binding of metformin to plasma proteins. This process is the opposite of what occurs with glyburide, which is cleared by the liver and kidneys with 99.8% bound to plasma proteins. Therefore, if metformin is used in pregnancy, its therapeutic level should be adjusted with the method of clearance due to the increased glomerular filtration rate in pregnancy. It is recommended that metformin be introduced gradually in 500- or 850-mg increments to a maximum effective dose of 2000 mg/daily. The absolute maximum dose is 2550 or 3000 mg/day. Administration in the presence of renal disease is contraindicated and requires caution [68,69].

At the cellular level, metformin improves insulin sensitivity. Its predominant glucose-lowering mechanism reduces the excessive rates of hepatic glucose production, which in turn reduces gluconeogenesis by increasing hepatic sensitivity to insulin. The drug also decreases hepatic glycogenolysis and increases insulin-stimulated glucose uptake in skeletal muscles. The cellular effects of metformin are to counteract insulin resistance and to reduce the acknowledged toxic metabolic effects of hyperglycemia (glucose toxicity) and fatty acids (lipotoxicity) in type 2 diabetes.

Clinical trials at two centers examined the effect of metformin as single therapy in nonpregnant obese subjects who had type 2 diabetes and in poorly controlled sulfonylurea-treated subjects. In both studies, the mean decline in plasma glucose concentration was approximatley 60 mg/dL, and beneficial effects on plasma lipid levels were observed [10,11,70].

Three frequently asked questions are: Should metformin for polycystic ovarian syndrome (PCO) be continued after patients become pregnant? Can metformin be used as a treatment modality in gestational diabetes? Should patients who have type 2 diabetes who achieved targeted levels of control with metformin remain on the drug or replace it with glyburide or insulin? To answer these questions, some issues need to be clarified: Does metformin cross the placenta? If it does, does it have a metabolic or teratogenic effect on the fetus? Most drugs used in pregnancy cross the placenta. However, few will cause adverse effects to the fetus.

Company information (Glucophage, Bristol-Myers Squibb, 1997) states that a partial placental barrier to metformin exists. Studies on transplacental transport of metformin demonstrated that it clearly crosses the placenta [71,72]. But, metformin has minimal affect on transplacental flux [37]. Of note, the transfer of metformin into human milk is minimal and, therefore, lactation in patients using metformin is not contraindicated [73,74].

The results of reproduction studies in rats and rabbits remain controversial. One study demonstrated no teratogenicity at doses up to 600 mg/kg/day, approximately twice the maximum recommended human dose on the basis of mg/m$^2$ [75]. Other studies have suggested that metformin induces a low incidence of malformations in rats [76,77]. In a more recent study, two-cell mouse embryos were exposed to different levels of metformin. Although lower levels comparable to plasma concentration during treatment did not affect the blastocyst development rate, the highest concentration resulted in a marked delay in development [78].

Because perfusion studies are difficult if not impossible to perform on a first-trimester placenta, and mice and rat placentas are not synonymous with human placentas (transfer in one does not mandate a transfer in the other), human studies evaluating the exposure to the drug during the first trimester and especially during organogenesis can supply the evidence for the efficacy of using certain drugs during pregnancy. However, randomized studies are unethical and, therefore, will never be endorsed during this gestational timeframe. The second best research design will be case-controlled and meta-analysis studies.

Several studies in the past decade have speculated that there was no association between oral hypoglycemic agents and congenital malformations. Notelowitz' [18] randomized study in 1971 treating patients with first generation sulfonylureas and insulin resulted in only two births with anomalies. One infant treated with tolbutamide had choanal atresia and the other, treated with insulin, had fallots syndrome. He concluded that sulfonylureas were safe for use in pregnancy. Towner and colleagues [79] treated 332 type 2 patients with oral hypoglycemic agents or insulin before pregnancy. They reported that the mode of therapy did not adversely affect the rate of anomalies, while glycemic levels as well as maternal age were significant contributing factors.

The author's practice described comparable findings in a retrospective analysis of 347 type 2 diabetic women exposed to different oral hypoglycemic agents, insulin, and diet therapy before and during the first trimester [80]. They demonstrated that the elevated blood glucose level and not the mode of therapy affected the rate of anomalies. Gilbert and Koren [81] presented a meta-analysis of all published studies with data on pregnancy outcome with respect to major malformations. The cohort included 72 PCOS patients who were exposed to metformin and compared with 48 PCOS patients who conceived without metformin in five different infertility clinics. They found no increase in the rate of malformations, and in fact, metformin might have had a protective effect (1.7% anomalies in the treated versus 7.2% in the untreated group). Recently, two studies reported the use of metformin in women who have polycystic ovary syndrome. Glueck and colleagues [82,83] suggested that metformin is safe and useful in the reduction of GDM in women who have PCOS. They evaluated 33 nondiabetic women who had PCOS who were treated with metformin prospectively and 39 nondiabetic women not treated with metformin evaluated retrospectively. The development of GDM was 3% in the former and 23% in the latter. In the second study, Jakubwicz and colleagues [84] sought to investigate the effect of preconceptual use of metformin on early pregnancy loss. They evaluated 65 women who had PCOS receiving metformin to 31 women not receiving the drug. The early pregnancy loss in the former was 11% and 58% in the untreated group. All 62 infants in the metformin-treated group were normal with the exception of 1 infant who had chondro-dysplasia. These two studies demonstrated that the use of metformin preconception and during the first trimester is not associated with major fetal malformations or fetal hypoglycemia after birth.

In summary, although metformin crosses the placenta, it is categorized as a class B drug. Its use in GDM is post first trimester, controlling against the risk of fetal anomalies (after the organogenesis period). From the current clinical data, it seems that it will be safe for the fetus (eg, macrosomia and hypoglycemia). This may be explained by its pharmacologic action to reduce hepatic glucose production and insulin resistance rather than pancreatic stimulation. Therefore, this drug may be a potentially attractive alternative to insulin in the management of patients who have GDM.

To date, no randomized study addressing the use of oral agents during organogenesis has been performed. However, the cumulative available data suggest that the cause of anomalies is the level of glycemia and not the use of oral hypoglycemic drugs. This is especially true since the first generation of sulfonylureas has been replaced by a second generation of oral hypoglycemic drugs. In summary, there is no justification to maintain a PCOS patient on metformin throughout pregnancy if she does not develop gestational diabetes. Most of the studies applicable to PCOS restricted metformin exposure to the first trimester; it was discontinued as soon as pregnancy was diagnosed. Evidence beyond the first trimester is anecdotal or based on small sample sizes. Until such time that a well-controlled study will be conducted in patients who have type 2 and GDM, its use should not be endorsed. We should await the results of ongoing randomized trials addressing the possible effect of metformin in pregnancy (eg, the Metformin in Gestational diabetes study) [85].

## Thiazolidenediones

To date, no study has reported data on the use of this group of drugs in pregnancy. The mechanism of action seems to reduce cellular insulin resistance by acting as a peroxisome proliferator-activated receptor. A decrease in systemic and local tissue lipid availability may also contribute to antidiabetic effects. In summary, the thiazolidenediones enter the cell and act within the nucleus (different than the sulfonylureas, which attach themselves to three different types of receptors on the cell membrane) by attaching to the peroxisome proliferator-activated receptor. They activate gene expression resulting in a cascade of cell signaling.

The pharmacokinetics of thiazolidenediones demonstrates that they are rapidly and almost completely absorbed 1 to 2 hours to peak concentration; absorption is slightly delayed when taken with food. The liver comprehensively metabolizes both drugs. Metabolism of rosiglitazone is mainly to weak active metabolites with lesser activity that are mostly eliminated in the urine; the metabolites of pioglitazone are more active and eliminated mostly in the bile. This group of drugs has similar characteristics to glyburide: they are bounded to plasma protein (99.8%) and have comparable molecular weights. The starting dosage for rosiglitazone is 4 mg/day and can be increased to 8 mg/day, once daily or in a divided dose. The drug can be given in combination therapy with metformin and/or sulfonylureas and/or insulin. Pioglitazone is administered once daily (15 mg) and can be increased to 30 mg and up to 45 mg as needed.

Thiazolidinediones are classified as pregnancy category C. These drugs should only be used during pregnancy if the potential benefit justifies the potential risk to the fetus. One needs to be cautious in the use of these drugs when there is evidence of liver disease or abnormal liver testing (alanine aminotransferase levels > 2.5 times the upper limit for the laboratory), and in patients who have heart disease or history of heart failure. Nevertheless, it is recommended that liver function be measured before initiation of therapy and bimonthly during the first year of treatment. There has been considerable weight gain reported with both drugs.

These contraindications are rare in pregnancy and, therefore, most patients will qualify for the use of the drug. Pregnancy is only one spectrum of the role of the obstetrician/gynecologist. Our mission is to address women's health overall. Thus, the obesity and metabolic syndrome epidemic, the PCOS which include approximately 20% of infertility cases, and the increased rate of gestational diabetes have created a large population of women who may benefit from metformin and the thiazolidilediones beyond the current benefits of glyburide (sulfonylureas).

Therefore, one can speculate that these drugs will not cross the placenta as is the case with glyburide and will allow us to use a potentially attractive drug because of its multisystemic response in gestational diabetes and in pregnancy in general. However, this wishful thinking is not the reality: these drugs cross the placenta. Several animal studies have demonstrated that these drugs cross the placental barrier and cause, in rats, delayed body growth and insulin resistance [86–88]. One study in vivo murine model found that rosiglitazone did not impair murine blastocyst development in vitro or cause phenotypic harm to the mouse fetus when administered during pregnancy [89]. These findings bring us back to the question previously addressed relevant to metformin: Is it enough to declare a drug contraindicated if the drug crosses the placenta or evidence of no damage to the embryo and fetus should permit us to use newly developed drugs with a potentially high benefit to the embryo, fetus, and mother?

Thiazolidenediones improve all body insulin sensitivity through multiple actions on gene regulation. The drugs enhance glucose uptake and disposal in the muscles. In the liver, there is improved insulin sensitivity and decreased gluconeogenesis. β-cell function in the pancreas is improved. The lipid profile is affected by pioglitazone with the reduction in triglyceride and an increased HDL and with rosiglitazone with decreased LDL and increased HDL. Adipose tissue is affected by increased GLUT4 expression, induced subcutaneous fat deposition, and decreased FFA release (reducing insulin resistance). Blood vessels demonstrate increased vasodilatation, decreased blood pressure, and vascular smooth muscle proliferation and migration, in addition to a reduction in inflammation (TNF)-$\alpha$. The homeostatic system shows a reduction in PA1-1 and fibrinogen as well as platelet aggregation. Therefore, the benefits of this group of drugs is beyond the glucose control of diabetes, but rather its contribution is multisystematic and may affect several component characteristics of the metabolic syndrome [90,91].

Troglitazone was the first thiazolidinedione marketed in the United States. However, after numerous reports of hepatotoxicity with the drug, followed by several deaths, it was voluntarily removed by the manufacturer in early March 2000. The second generation of these drugs (ie, rosiglitazone and pioglitazone) are more potent and have not shown the hepatotoxicity found in troglitazone [92]. Studies in prediabetic animal models suggest that treatment with thiazolidineiones may be capable of preventing diabetes progression and pancreatic exhaustion and of protecting against nephropathy. In the diabetic model, control of blood glucose by this drug was accompanied by pancreatic recovery and normalization of pancreatic insulin storage and synthesis [93,94].

In humans, one study suggested that in women who had previous gestational diabetes, troglitazone reduced the incidence of new onset diabetes [95]. If the second generation of drugs in this group proves to be more effective, than antidiabetic agents currently in use to reduce the decline in $\beta$-cell function in patients who have type 2 diabetes still needs to be determined [96]. A recent double-blind randomized controlled clinical trial of 4360 women recently diagnosed with type 2 diabetes evaluated the potential risk/benefit of monotherapy failure at 5 years of three different drugs. The primary outcome was the time to monotherapy failure, which was defined as a confirmed level of fasting plasma glucose of greater than 180 mg/dL. This is another example of different levels of success in therapy that are used in pregnancy and nonpregnancy. Therefore, different considerations must be addressed in pregnancy. The failure rate with rosiglitazone was 15%, 21% with metformin, and 34% with glyburide [97]. Finally, it was shown in overweight and obese patients who had impaired glucose tolerance who were younger that after 3 years of treatment with metformin, the incidence of type 2 diabetes decreased by 33% and that an intensive regimen of diet and exercise alone reduced the risk by 58% (major lifestyle change) [98].

### $\alpha$-Glucosidase inhibitors

Drugs in this class act by slowing the absorption of carbohydrates from the intestines thus minimizing the postprandial rise in blood glucose [99].

Gastrointestinal side effects require gradual dosage increments, over weeks to months, after initiation of therapy. Acarbose, miglitol, and voglibose, currently in clinical use, may be added to most other available therapies [100,101]. The α-glucosidase inhibitors do not cause weight gain, they reduce postprandial hyperinsulinemia, and they *may* lower plasma triglyceride levels. These drugs reduce postprandial glucose levels by 1 to 4 mmol/L. The area under the curve (of the post meal) may be reduced by half, while the basal glycemia may be reduced by up to 1 mmol/L. HbA1c decreases by 0.5% to 1% [102]. The experience in pregnancy is minimal with fewer than 100 patients to date. This is despite the fact that acarbose acts within the gastrointestinal tract and is not transferred by the blood stream to the placenta. However, its ability to decrease glucose to targeted levels required in pregnancy is less effective than glyburide [103]. Therefore, it is less effective than glyburide; its use in pregnancy should be confined to combinations with glyburide and possibly metformin rather than monotherapy.

## Summary

Different oral hypoglycemic agents act upon different mechanisms of action. For patients who have newly diagnosed type 2 diabetes without markedly elevated plasma fasting glucose (eg, > 280 mg/dL), it is advisable to begin oral therapy with monotherapy such as glyburide or probably metformin. Glyburide is currently the only drug shown to not cross the placenta and studied clinically in properly designed randomized controlled trials. However, other oral hypoglycemic agents may have an even greater therapeutic effect on glycemic levels and other metabolic complications.

The achievement of both glucose and outcome goals is conditional upon the overall successful management of women who have GDM. This will include appropriate caloric as well as meal/snack allotment throughout the day, verified self-monitoring of blood glucose, proper criteria for initiation of the drug, and education/behavior modification for the patient. Failure to address any of these components of intensified therapy will compromise the success rate of glucose control and, in turn, the perinatal outcome. The control of glucose and not the drug is the key to success.

## References

[1] US Preventive Services Task Force. Agency for Healthcare Research and Quality. Department of Health and Human Services; Bulletin 1996.
[2] Reaven GM. The role of insulin resistance in human disease. Diabetes 1998;37:1595–607.
[3] Olefsky JM. Pathogenesis of non-insulin dependent diabetes (type 2). In: DeGroot LJ, Nesser GM, Cahill JC, editors. Endocrinology. 2nd edition. Philadelphia: WB Saunders; 1989. p. 1369–88.
[4] Langer O. Maternal glycemic criteria for insulin therapy in gestational diabetes mellitus. Diabetes Care 1998;21(Suppl 2):B91–8.

[5] Schade DS, Jovanovic L, Schneider J. A placebo-controlled randomized study of glimepiride in patients with type 2 diabetes mellitus for whom diet therapy is unsuccessful. J Clin Pharmacol 1998;38:636–41.

[6] Langer O, Conway DL, Berkus MD, et al. A comparison glyburide and insulin in women with gestational diabetes mellitus. N Engl J Med 2000;343(16):1134–8.

[7] Langer O, Rodriguez DA, Xenakis EMJ, et al. Intensified vs.conventional management of gestational diabetes. Am J Obstet Gynecol 1994;170:1036–47.

[8] Langer O, Yogev Y, Xenakis E, et al. Overweight and obese in gestational diabetes: the impact on pregnancy outcome. Am J Obstet Gynecol 2005;192(6):1768–76.

[9] McFarland MB, Langer O, Conway DL, et al. Dietary therapy for gestational diabetes: how long enough? Obstet Gynecol 1999;93:978–82.

[10] American Diabetes Association. Implications of the United Kingdom Prospective Diabetes Study. Diabetes Care 2000;23(Suppl 2):S27–31.

[11] Anonymous. The effects of intensive treatment of diabetes on the development and progression of long-term complications in insulin-dependent diabetes mellitus. N Engl J Med 1993; 329:977–86.

[12] Douglas CP, Richards R. Use of chlorpropamide in the treatment of diabetes in pregnancy. Diabetes 1967;16:60–1.

[13] Jackson WPU, Campbell GD, Notelowitz M, et al. Tolbutamide and chloroprompamide during pregnancy in human diabetics. Diabetes 1962;11(Suppl):98–101.

[14] Sutherland HW, Bewsher PD, Cormack JD, et al. Effect of moderate dosage of chloropropamide in pregnancy on fetal outcome. Arch Dis Child 1974;149:283–91.

[15] Coetzee EJ, Jackson WPU. Oral hypoglycemics in the first trimester and fetal outcome. S Afr Med J 1984;65:635–7.

[16] Coetzee EJ, Jackson WPU. Pregnancy in established non-insulin-dependent diabetics. S Afr Med J 1980;61:795–802.

[17] Notelowitz M. Oral hypoglycemic therapy in diabetic pregnancies. Lancet 1974;2:902–3.

[18] Notelowitz M. Sulfonylurea therapy in the treatment of the pregnant diabetic. S Afr Med J 1971;45:226–9.

[19] Coetzee EJ, Jackson WPU. The management of non-insulin-dependent diabetes during pregnancy. Diabetes Res Clin Pract 1986;1:281–7.

[20] Coetzee EJ. Oral hypoglycemic agents in the treatment of gestational diabetes. In: Jovanovic L, editor. Endocrinology and metabolism controversies in diabetes and pregnancy. Berlin: Springer-Verlag; 1988. p. 57–76.

[21] Coetzee EJ, Jackson WPU. Metformin in management of pregnant insulin-independent diabetics. Diabetologia 1979;16:241–5.

[22] Steel JM, Johnstone FD. Sulphonylureas in pregnancy. Lancet 1991;338:1122.

[23] American Diabetes Association. Gestational diabetes mellitus. American Diabetes Association: clinical practice recommendations. Diabetes Care 1998;21:S60–1.

[24] Metzger BE, Coustan DR, , the organizing committee. Summary and recommendations of the fourth international workshop conference on gestational diabetes. Diabetes Care 1998; 21(Suppl 2):B161–7.

[25] American College of Obstetricians and Gynecologists. Management of diabetes mellitus in pregnancy. Technical Bulletin 92. Washington, DC: ACOG; 1996. p. 1–2.

[26] Kemball ML, McIvert C, Milner RDG, et al. Neonatal hypoglycemia in infants of diabetic mothers given sulphonylurea drugs in pregnancy. Arch Dis Child 1970;45: 696–701.

[27] Farquar JW, Isles TE. Hypoglycemia in newborn infants of normal and diabetic mothers. S Afr Med J 1968;9:237–45.

[28] Zucker P, Simon G. Prolonged symptomatic neonatal hypoglycemia associated with maternal chlorpropamide therapy. Pediatrics 1968;42:824–5.

[29] Piacquadio K, Hollingsworth DR, Murphy H. Effects of in-utero exposure to oral hypoglycemic drugs. Lancet 1991;338:866–9.

[30] Groop L, Luzi L, Melanger A, et al. Different effects of glyburide and glipizide on insulin secretion and hepatic glucose production in normal and NIDDM subjects. Diabetes 1987; 36:1320–8.

[31] Groop LC, Barzilai N, Ratheiser K, et al. Dose-dependent effects of glyburide on insulin secretion and glucose uptake in humans. Diabetes Care 1991;14:724–7.

[32] DeFronzo RA, Simonson DC. Oral sulfonylurea agents suppress hepatic glucose production in non-insulin-dependent diabetic individuals. Diabetes Care 1984;7:72–80.

[33] Rossetti L, Giaaccari A, DeFronzo RA. Glucose toxicity. Diabetes Care 1990;13:610–30.

[34] Simonson DC, Farrannini E, Bevilacqua S, et al. Mechanism of improvement in glucose metabolism after chronic glyburide therapy. Diabetes Care 1984;33:838–45.

[35] Elliot B, Langer O, Schenker S, et al. Insignificant transfer of glyburide occurs across the human placenta. Am J Obstet Gynecol 1991;165:807–12.

[36] Elliot B, Schenker S, Langer O, et al. Comparative placental transport of oral hypoglycemic agents: a model of human placental drug transfer. Am J Obstet Gynecol 1994;171: 653–60.

[37] Elliot B, Langer O, Schussling F. A model of human placental drug transfer. Am J Obstet Gynecol 1997;176:527–30.

[38] Koren G. Glyburide and fetal safety: transplacental pharmacokinetic considerations. Reprod Toxicol 2001;15:227–9.

[39] Nanovskaya TN, Nekhayeva I, Hankins G, et al. Effect of human serum albumin on transplacental transfer of glyburide. Biochem Pharmacol 2006;72:632–9.

[40] Kraemer J, Klein J, Lubetsky A, et al. Perfusion studies of glyburide transfer across the human placenta: implications for fetal safety. Am J Obstet Gynecol 2006;195:270–4.

[41] Langer O. Oral hypoglycemic agents and the pregnant diabetic: "From bench to bedside". Semin Perinatol 2002;26(3):215–24.

[42] Langer O. Oral hypoglycemic agents in pregnancy: their time has come. J Matern Fetal Neonatal Med 2002;12:376–83.

[43] Langer O. Gestational diabetes and oral hypoglycemic agents: a fresh look at the safety profile. OBG Management 2003;15(8):62–76.

[44] Langer O. Management of gestational diabetes: pharmacologic treatment options and glycemic control. Endocrinol Metab Clin North Am 2006;35:53–78.

[45] Langer O. The diabetes in pregnancy dilemma: leading change with proven solutions. Lanham, Maryland: University Press of America; 2006.

[46] Bailey CJ, Day C. Antidiabetic drugs. Br J Cardiol 2003;10:128–36.

[47] DeFronzo RA. Pharmacologic therapy for type 2 diabetes mellitus. Ann Intern Med 1999; 131:281–303.

[48] Langer O, Conway DL. Level of glycemia and perinatal outcome in pregestational diabetes. J Matern Fetal Med 2001;9(1):35–41.

[49] Langer O. A spectrum of glucose thresholds may effectively prevent complications in the pregnant diabetic patient. Semin Perinatol 2002;26(3):196–205.

[50] Langer O. Is normoglycemia the correct threshold to prevent complications in the pregnant diabetic? Diabetic Rev 1996;4(1):2–10.

[51] Chmait R, Dinise T, Daneshmand S, et al. Prospective cohort study to establish predictors of glyburide success in gestational diabetes mellitus. J Perinatol 2004 Oct;24(10):617–22.

[52] Hellmuth E, Damm P, Molsted-Pedersen L. Oral hypoglycemic agents in 118 diabetic pregnancies. Diabet Med 2000;17(7):507–11.

[53] Lim JM, Tayob Y, O'brien PM, et al. A comparison between the pregnancy outcome of women with gestation diabetes treated with glibenclamide and those treated with insulin. Med J Malaysia 1997;52(4):377–81.

[54] Conway DL, Gonzales O, Skiver D. Use of glyburide for the treatment of gestational diabetes: the San Antonio experience. J Matern Fetal Neonatal Med 2004;15(1):51–5.

[55] Kremer CJ, Duff P. Glyburide for the treatment of gestational diabetes. Am J Obstet Gynecol 2004;190(5):1438–9.

[56] Chmait R, Dinise T, Moore T. Prospective observational study to establish predictors of glyburide success in women with gestational diabetes mellitus. J Perinatol 2004 Oct;24(10): 617–22.

[57] Gilson G, Murphy N. Comparison of oral glyburide with insulin for the management of gestational diabetes mellitus in Alaskan native women. Am J Obstet Gynecol 2002 Dec; 187(6, part 2) Suppl:S152, A336.

[58] Fines V, Moore T, Castle S. A comparison of glyburide and insulin treatment in gestational diabetes mellitus on infant birth weight and adiposity. Am J Obstet Gynecol 2003 Dec; 189(6) Suppl 1:S108, A161.

[59] Velazquez MD, Bolnick J, Cloakey D. The use of glyburide in the management of gestational diabetes. Obstet Gynecol 2003;101(4 Suppl):88S.

[60] Pendsey SP, Sharma RR, Chalkhore SS. Repaglinde: a feasible alternative to insulin in management of gestational diabetes mellitus. Diabetes Res Clin Pract 2002;56Suppl1: S44–45, OR103.

[61] Jacobson GF, Ramos GA, Ching JY, et al. Comparison of glyburide and insulin for the management of gestational diabetes in a large managed care organization. Am J Obstet Gynecol 2005;193(1):118–24.

[62] UKPDS (UK Prospective Diabetes Study). Intensive blood-glucose control with sulphonylurea or insulin compared with conventional treatment and risk of complications in patients with type 2 diabetes (UPDS 33). Lancet 1998;352:837–53.

[63] Harris MI, Eastman RC, Cowie CC, et al. Racial and ethnic differences in glycemic control of adults with type 2 diabetes. Diabetes Care 1999;22(3):403–8.

[64] Liebl A, Mata M, Eschwege E. ODE-2 Advisory Board. Evaluation of risk factors for development of complications in type II diabetes in Europe. Diabetologia 2002;45(7): S23–8.

[65] Yogev Y, Ben-Haroush A, Chen R, et al. Undiagnosed asymptomatic hypoglycemia: diet, insulin, and glyburide for gestational diabetic pregnancy. Obstet Gynecol 2004; 104:88–93.

[66] Bailey CJ, Turner RC. Metformin. N Engl J Med 1996;334:574–9.

[67] Krentz AJ, Bailey CJ. Oral antidiabetic agents: current role in type 2 diabetes mellitus. Drugs 2005;65(3):385–411.

[68] Kirpichnikov D, McFarlene SI, Sower JR. Metformin: an update. Ann Intern Med 2002; 137:25–33.

[69] Cuzi K, DeFronzo RA. Metformin: a review of its metabolic effects. Diabetes Rev 1998;6: 89–131.

[70] Turner RC, Cull CA, Fright V, et al. Glycemic control with diet, sulfonylurea, metformin, or insulin in patients with type 2 diabetes mellitus: Progressive requirement for multiple therapies. J Am Med Assoc 1999;281:2005–12.

[71] Nanovskaya TN, Nekhayeva IA, Patrikeeva SL, et al. Transfer of metformin across the dually perfused human placental lobule. Am J Obstet Gynecol 2006;195:1081–5.

[72] Kovo N, Haroutiunian S, Feldman N, et al. Determination of metformin transfer across the human placenta using dually perfused ex-vivo placental cotyledon model [abstract]. Am J Obstet Gynecol 2005;193(6):S85.

[73] Hale TW, Kristensen JH, Hacket LP, et al. Transfer of metformin into human milk. Diabetologia 2002;45:1509–14.

[74] Gardiner SJ, Kirkpatrick CM, Begg EJ, et al. Transfer of metformin into human milk. Clin Pharmacol Ther 2003;73:71–7.

[75] Briggs GG, Freeman RK, Yaffe SJ. Drugs in pregnancy and lactation. Philadelphia: Lippincott, Williams and Wilkins; 2002. p. 270.

[76] Shepard TH. Catalog of teratogenic agents. 8th edition. Baltimore (MD): John Hopkins University Press; 1995.

[77] Schardein JL. Chemically induced birth defects. 2nd edition. New York: Marcel Dekker; 1993. p. 417–8.

[78] Bedaiwy MA, Miller KF, Goldberg JM, et al. Effect of metformin on mouse embryo development. Fertil Steril 2001;76:1078–9.
[79] Towner D, Kjos SL, Montoro MM, et al. Congenital malformations in pregnancies complicated by NIDDM. Diabetes Care 1995;18(11):1446–51.
[80] Langer O, Conway D, Berkus M, et al. There is no association between hypoglycemic use and fetal anomalies [abst]. Am J Obstet Gynecol 1999;180(1):S38.
[81] Gilbert C, Koren G. Pregnancy outcome following first-trimester exposure to metformin: a meta-analysis [abstract]. Can J Pharmacol 2005;12(1):e125.
[82] Glueck CJ, Wang P, Kobayashi S, et al. Metformin therapy throughout pregnancy reduces the development of gestational diabetes in women with polycystic ovary syndrome. Fertil Steril 2002;77:520–5.
[83] Glueck CJ, Goldenberg N, Wang P, et al. Metformin during pregnancy reduces insulin, insulin resistance, insulin secretion, weight, testosterone and development of gestational diabetes: prospective longitudinal assessment of women with polycystic ovary syndrome from preconception throughout pregnancy. Hum Reprod 2004;19(3):510–21.
[84] Jakubwicz DJ, Iuorno MJ, Jakubowicz S, et al. Effects of metformin on early pregnancy loss in the polycystic ovary syndrome. J Clin Endocrinol Metab 2002;87:524–8.
[85] Hague WM, Davoren PM, Oliver J, et al. Contraindications to use metformin: metformin may be useful in gestational diabetes. Br Med J 2003 Apr 5;326(7392):762.
[86] Sevillano J, Lopez-Perez IC, Herrera E, et al. Englitazone administration to late pregnant rats produces delayed body growth and insulin resistance in their fetuses and neonates. Biochem J 2005;389:913–8.
[87] Chan LYS, Yeung JH, Lau TK. Placental transfer of rosiglitazone in the first trimester of human pregnancy. Fertil Steril 2005;83(4):955–8.
[88] Wareing M, Greenwood SL, Fyfe GK, et al. Glibenclamide inhibits agonist-induced vasoconstriction of placental chorionic plate arteries. Placenta 2006;27:660–8.
[89] Klinker DR, Lim HJ, Strawn EY, et al. An in vivo murine model of rosiglitazone use in pregnancy. Fertil Steril 2006;86(Suppl 3):1074–9.
[90] Day C. Thiazolidinediones: a new class of anti-diabetic drugs. Diabet Med 1999;16:1–14.
[91] Yki-Jarvinen H. Thiazolidinedions. N Engl J Med 2004;351:1106–18.
[92] Krentz AJ, Bailey CJ, Melander A. Thiazolidinediones for type 2 diabetes. BMJ 2000;321:252–3.
[93] Buckingham RE, AL-Barazanji KA, Toseland N, et al. Peroxisome proliferator-activated receptor-gamma agonist, rosiglitazone, protects against nephropathy and pancreatic islet abnormalities in Zucker fatty rats. Diabetes 1998;47:1326–34.
[94] Lebovitz HE. Thiazolidinediones. In: Lebovitz HE, editor. Therapy for diabetes mellitus and related disorders. 3rd edition. Alexandria (VA): American Diabetes Association; 1998. p. 181–5.
[95] Buchanan TA, Xiang AH, Peters RK, et al. Preservation of pancreatic beta-cell function and prevention of type 2 diabetes by pharmacological treatment of insulin in high-risk Hispanic women. Diabetes 2002;51:2796–803.
[96] Bell DS. Beta-cell rejuvenation with thiazolidenediones. Am J Med 2003 Dec 8;115Suppl 8A:20S–23S.
[97] Kahn SE, Haffner SM, Heise MA, et al. Glycemic durability of rosiglitazone, metformin or glyburide monotherapy. N Engl J Med 2006;355:2427–43.
[98] Diabetes Prevention Program Research Group. Reduction of the incidence of type 2 diabetes with lifestyle intervention or metformin. N Engl J Med 2002;346:393–403.
[99] Lebovitz HE. α-Glucosidase inhibitors as agents in the treatment of diabetes. Diabetes Revs 1998;6:132–45.
[100] Coniff RF, Seaton TB, Shapiro JA, et al. Reduction of glycosylated hemoglobin and postprandial hyperglycemia by acarbose in patients with NIDDM. Diabetes Care 1995;18:817–20.
[101] Lebovitz HE. α-Glucosidas inhibitors. Endocrinol Metab Clin North Am 1997;26:539–51.

[102] Holman RR, Cull CA, Turner RC. A randomized double-blind trial of acarbose in type 2 diabetes shows improved glycemic control over 3 years (UK Prospective Diabetes Study 44).
Diabetes Care 1999;22:960–4.
[103] Bertini AM, Silva JC, Taborda W, et al. Perinatal outcomes and the use of oral hypoglycemic agents. J Perinat Med 2005;33:519–23.

ELSEVIER
SAUNDERS

Obstet Gynecol Clin N Am
34 (2007) 275–291

OBSTETRICS AND
GYNECOLOGY
CLINICS
OF NORTH AMERICA

# Insulin Analogues in the Treatment of Diabetes in Pregnancy

## Charanpal Singh, MD, Lois Jovanovic, MD

*Sansum Diabetes Research Institute, 2219 Bath Street, Santa Barbara, CA 93105, USA*

Before the advent of insulin in 1922, less than 100 pregnancies in diabetic women were reported; most likely these women had type 2 and not type 1 diabetes [1]. Even with this assumption, these cases of diabetes and pregnancy were associated with a greater than 90% infant mortality rate and a 30% maternal mortality rate. As late as 1980, physicians were still counseling diabetic women to avoid pregnancy. This philosophy was justified because of the poor obstetric history in 30% to 50% of diabetic women. Improved infant mortality rates finally occurred after 1980, when treatment strategies stressed better control of maternal plasma glucose levels, once self-blood glucose monitoring and glycosylated hemoglobin became available. As the pathophysiology of pregnancy complicated by diabetes has been elucidated and as management programs have achieved and maintained near normoglycemia throughout pregnancy complicated by diabetes mellitus, perinatal mortality rates have decreased to levels seen in the general population [2–9]. This review reports the literature on the safety and efficacy of insulin analogues in pregnancy and thereby enables the clinician to choose the optimal insulin treatment protocol to achieve and maintain normoglycemia throughout pregnancies complicated by diabetes.

## Rationale for the use of nonimmunogenic insulins during pregnancy

Maternal glucose freely crosses the placenta. Maternal insulin does not cross the placenta unless it is bound to IgG antibody, which carries it through the placenta, or insulin is forced through the placenta by high perfusion [10,11]. Diabetic fetopathy is thought to be the result of fetal hyperinsulinemia [1–9]. Thus treatment must be designed to normalize maternal blood glucose concentrations without the use of exogenous insulins that

---

*E-mail address:* ljovanovic@sansum.org (L. Jovanovic).

doi:10.1016/j.ogc.2007.03.003                                    *obgyn.theclinics.com*

cross the placenta. Placental transfer of insulin complexed with immuno-globulin has also been associated with fetal macrosomia in mothers who have near-normal glycemic control during gestation. Menon and colleagues [12] reported that antibody-bound insulin transferred to the fetus was proportional to the concentration of antibody-bound insulin measured in the mother. Also, the amount of antibody-bound insulin transferred to the fetus correlated directly with macrosomia in the infant and was independent of maternal blood glucose levels. In contrast, Jovanovic and colleagues [13] discovered that it was only improved glucose control, as evidenced by lower postprandial glucose excursions, but not lower insulin antibody levels, correlated with lower fetal weight. They showed that insulin antibodies to exogenous insulin do not influence infant birth weight.

The literature is now well documented that maintenance of postprandial glucose concentrations in the normal range decreases the risk of glucose-mediated macrosomia [6–8]. Rapid-acting insulin analogues have been shown to improve postprandial glucose control compared with the concentrations resulting from treatment with human regular insulin. Data [14] suggest that rapid-acting insulin analogues do not transfer through the human placenta, thus they can be considered suitable therapeutic candidates as treatment during pregnancies complicated by diabetes [10,11,15–20]. However, to date, the clinical data currently available for the long-acting insulin analogues is not sufficient to advocate their use in pregnancy. This article reviews the literature on the insulin analogue during pregnancy and presents the authors' opinion as to the safety and efficacy of insulin analogue treatment for the pregnant diabetic woman.

## Insulin therapy during pregnancy

The anti-insulin hormones from the placenta along with an increased maternal cortisol concentration in concert with increasing weight gain and decreasing exercise result in a rise in insulin requirement. The 24-hour insulin requirement before conception is approximately 0.8 units times the mother's weight in kilograms. In the first trimester, the insulin requirement rises to 0.7 units per kilogram times the pregnant weight of the woman. By the second trimester, the insulin requirement is 0.8 units per kilogram; by term, the insulin requirement is 0.9 times 1.0 unit per kilogram pregnant weight per day [21]. There is a transient drop of insulin requirement in the first trimester, however [22]. During first trimester, the placental passage of glucose and gluconeogenic along with the luteoplacental shift of progesterone from the corpus luteum to the placenta with a transient drop in progesterone levels work in concert to decrease the insulin requirement in the late-third first trimester; substrates may cause maternal hypoglycemia if the doses of insulin are not decreased by 10%. In addition, blood glucose control during this period is also more unstable, with a tendency to low fasting plasma glucose and high postprandial excursions and the occurrence of nocturnal hypoglycemia. Lastly, pregnancy-induced nausea and vomiting can predispose to hypoglycemia. During the second and third trimesters, the progressively increased production of placental anti-insulin hormones causes progressive increments in insulin requirements; from the 24th gestational week, there is tendency to decrease in glucose excursions. In the last month of pregnancy, there may be a decrease in insulin requirement, particularly during the night because of transfer of maternal glucose and amino acid through placenta to the fetus, which accelerates growth [23].

All these metabolic characteristics lead to a greater demand for short-acting insulin, which covers the meal, and the need to optimize doses of intermediate-acting insulin, to guarantee a constant basal rate [24–34]. In this context, the special characteristics of the new insulins currently on the market can considerably help in the attainment of the desired metabolic control level during pregnancy. There are three rapid-acting insulins currently available on the market: insulin lispro, insulin aspart, and insulin glulisine. The two long-acting insulin analogues are insulin glargine and insulin detemir.

### Rapid-acting insulin analogues commercially available

Insulin lispro was first approved in 1996. It is the result of recombinant DNA technology and modifies the beta-chain of human insulin by inverting the position of lysine from B29 to B28 with that of proline from B28 to B29. This insulin is quickly dissociated into monomeric subunits when injected into subcutaneous tissue; it shows rapid action due to more rapid absorption through capillary membrane compared with insulin, and its use of insulin lispro is associated with a 27 to 36 mg/dL (1.5–2.0 mmol/L) lower postprandial glucose concentration ($P < .001$), improvement in hemoglobin $A_{1c}$ (A1C) of 0.3 to 0.5% points, and reduction of hypoglycemia rate by 20 to 30% ($P < .0024$) [35–39].

Insulin aspart, approved for clinical use in 1999, is created by replacing proline in B28 position with the negatively charged aspartic acid. The rapid dissociation into monomers occurs because of charge repulsion in the tertiary structure. The onset of insulin aspart is from 5 to 15 minutes of injection and peaks from 31 to 70 minutes after injection, with a duration of action from 2 to 4 hours. In comparison with regular insulin, insulin aspart reduces values of postprandial plasma glucose by approximately 27 mg/dL (1.5 mmol/L) ($P < .001$), A1C by 0.12% ($P < .02$), and serious hypoglycemic episodes by 50% ($P < .005$) [40–43].

### Insulin glulisine

Insulin glulisine is a rapid-acting human insulin analogue that has a faster onset of action and shorter duration of action than regular human insulin in patients who have type 1 or 2 diabetes mellitus and is efficacious in controlling prandial blood glucose levels in these patients. In large, well-designed trials in patients who had type 1 diabetes, insulin glulisine demonstrated a similar degree of glycemic control, as measured by glycosylated hemoglobin A1C levels, to regular human insulin after 12 weeks and insulin lispro after 26 weeks. Premeal insulin glulisine was also more effective than regular human insulin at controlling 2-hour postprandial glucose excursions in patients who had type 1 or 2 diabetes over a period of 12 weeks. In patients who had type 2 diabetes, insulin glulisine induced significantly greater reductions in hemoglobin A1C levels and 2-hour postbreakfast and postdinner blood glucose levels than regular human insulin over a period of 26 weeks. Insulin glulisine was generally well tolerated by patients who had type 1 or 2 diabetes and had a similar safety profile to insulin lispro or regular human insulin. Severe hypoglycemia was experienced by similar proportions of insulin glulisine or comparator insulin (insulin lispro or regular human insulin) recipients who had type 1 or type 2 diabetes [44,45]. There are no clinical trials to date using insulin glulisine, and thus no clinical recommendation can be made [46].

## Rapid-acting insulins in the treatment of diabetes and pregnancy

### Insulin lispro

The first randomized study that evaluated the effect of insulin lispro treatment in pregnancy was that of Jovanovic and colleagues [20], in which 19 patients on lispro who had gestational diabetes mellitus (GDM) and 23 on regular insulin were studied. In patients on lispro, the number of maternal hypoglycemic episodes before breakfast (plasma glucose < 55 mg/dL) was 24% lower than those of patients in regular insulin. The number of episodes of postprandial hyperglycemia (1-hour plasma glucose > 120 mg/dL) was also significantly lower in patients on insulin lispro than those on regular insulin. Moreover, treatment with lispro caused a significantly greater reduction in A1C levels at the third trimester in treatment group given lispro versus the group given regular insulin [47].

In a subsequent paper, Bhattacharyya and colleagues [48] evaluated 68 women who had GDM treated with insulin lispro and 89 with regular insulin; a significant reduction in A1C levels was found in patients on lispro with respect to those on regular insulin at the third trimester of pregnancy. The mean dose of short-acting insulin was similar in the two groups of patients. At the same time, patients on lispro reported greater satisfaction with treatment. Meccaci and colleagues [49] compared glucose levels and neonatal outcome in 49 women who had GDM randomly assigned to treatment with regular insulin and insulin lispro. Both types of insulin resulted good outcome and did not have significantly differing glycemic levels prepandially. Moreover, blood glucose values at the 1-hour postprandial point were significantly lower in patients on insulin lispro than in those on regular insulin. There was no statistical significant difference between the groups in neonatal outcome, though the number of neonates with a cranial/thoracic circumference ratio between 10th and 25th percentiles was higher in the group on the regular insulin. These results show that in women who have GDM, insulin lispro can normalize 1-hour postprandial glucose concentrations and is associated with normal anthropometric characteristics in the neonates.

The study reported by Wyatt and colleagues [50] was designed to determine the rate of congenital anomalies in offspring of women who have type 1 diabetes treated by insulin lispro before and during at least the first 12 weeks of gestation. This multinational, multicenter retrospective study included mothers who had diabetes mellitus (diagnosed before conception) who were treated with insulin lispro for at least 1 month before conception and during at least the first trimester of pregnancy. Anomalies were assessed by two independent dysmorphologists. The charts of 496 women were reviewed for 533 pregnancies resulting in 542 offspring (500 live births, 31 spontaneous and 7 elective abortions, and 4 stillbirths). Mothers' characteristics: mean ($\pm$ standard deviation [SD]) age was 29.9 ($\pm$ 5.2) years, 85.6% were Caucasian, and 97.2% had type 1 diabetes mellitus. Insulin lispro continued to be the main mealtime insulin for more than 96% of the women during the second and third trimester. The dysmorphologists determined that 27 (5.4%) offspring had major congenital anomalies and 2 (0.4%) offspring had minor congenital anomalies. The rate of major congenital anomalies was 5.4% [95% confidence interval (3.45%, 7.44%)] for offspring of mothers who had diabetes mellitus treated with insulin lispro before and during pregnancy. The current published rates of major anomalies in infants born to mothers who have diabetes treated with insulin are between 2.1% and 10.9%. This suggests that the anomaly rate with insulin lispro treatment does not differ from the published major congenital anomaly rates for other insulin treatments.

The other major study to evaluate glycemic control and maternal and fetal outcomes of patients who have type 1 diabetes treated with lispro before and during pregnancy was reported by Garg and colleagues [51]. They reviewed the medical records of 62 patients who had type 1 diabetes treated with insulin lispro. The mean A1C level reduced from $7.2 \pm 0.2\%$ at conception to $5.8 \pm 0.1\%$ at the time of delivery. No significant change was found in mean eye grade score for retinopathy or in albumin excretion rate during pregnancy. The mean duration of gestation was 37 weeks, and 24% of pregnancies resulting in neonatal macrosomia.

*Insulin aspart*

Currently, there are limited results regarding use of insulin aspart during pregnancy. Pettitt and colleagues [52] conducted the first clinical study to compare the short-term efficacy of insulin aspart, regular insulin, or no insulin in patients who have GDM. Fifteen women who had GDM received a standard meal test after administration of regular insulin or insulin aspart on 3 consecutive days (1 day was untreated baseline). Insulin aspart was administered 5 minutes before the meal, whereas regular insulin was administered 30 minutes before the meal. The postprandial glycemic control (as measured by glucose area under the curve above baseline) was significantly improved by insulin aspart compared with no exogenous insulin administered, whereas regular insulin did not show a significant difference from no exogenous insulin administered. These same investigators then observed a sample size of 27 women randomized to either receive insulin aspart or regular insulin for prandial treatment of their carbohydrate intolerance [52,53]. Both treatment groups maintained good overall glycemic control during the study. Insulin aspart was effective in reducing the postprandial glucose concentration from baseline. The contribution of endogenous insulin to the overall insulin profile was ascertained by measurement of the C-peptide values. C-peptide values for both insulin aspart and regular insulin treatments were slightly lower at week 6 than at week 0. However, insulin aspart treatment showed significantly lower C-peptide values at week 0 and week 6 than regular insulin as demonstrated by the significantly greater reduction in the change-from-baseline C-peptide values. No major hypoglycemic events were reported in this study. Antibody binding specific to insulin aspart and regular insulin remained low (less than 1.5% binding of the specific antibodies) for both treatment groups throughout the study. Cord blood serum samples, collected immediately after delivery, only detected raised levels of insulin (ether aspart or human regular insulin) if high infusion rates of insulin and glucose were administered during labor and delivery [52]. The neonatal birth weights were similar in both groups, and no case of macrosomia was reported. These studies demonstrate that the overall safety and effectiveness of insulin aspart was comparable to regular human insulin in pregnant women who have GDM. Insulin aspart was more effective than regular human insulin in providing postprandial glycemic control in women who have GDM.

Hod [53] recently presented the study design for a large multinational, multicenter randomized clinical trial observing the safety and efficacy of insulin aspart for the treatment of type 1 diabetes. This trial in 17 countries at 90 centers randomized 330 women who had type 1 diabetes to receive either human regular insulin or insulin aspart. This trial will be completed by the end of 2008. Thus far there have been no insulin-associated maternal or fetal complications, and no evidence that insulin aspart is teratogenic.

There are no clinical trials using insulin glulisine, and thus there no clinical recommendations that can be made [44–46]. However, based on the data for insulin lispro and insulin aspart, these two rapid-acting insulin analogues are safe and efficacious premeal insulin for use by pregnant diabetic women requiring mealtime insulin. Because of the rapid-acting analogues' favorable pharmacokinetics, postprandial blood glucose concentrations are improved compared with human regular insulin or no insulin treatment and thus may be considered as a treatment choice for pregnant diabetic women. Table 1 summarizes the 12 published articles to date [20,48–58] that report on 1425 pregnant diabetic women (1150 type 1 diabetic women and 275 gestational diabetic women), of whom 795 were treated with insulin lispro during pregnancy and 59 were treated with insulin aspart during pregnancy. Although not all reports were compared with outcome of pregnancy with human regular insulin treatment, the overall conclusion is that insulin lispro

Table 1
Use of rapid-acting insulin analogues in pregnancy

| Studies | Number | Type of DM | Lispro | Aspart | Regular | Outcome |
|---|---|---|---|---|---|---|
| Jovanovic et al [20] | 42 | GDM | 19 | 0 | 23 | ↓ pp with lispro |
| Bhattacharyya et al [48] | 157 | GDM | 68 | 0 | 89 | ↓ A1C levels with lispro |
| Mecacci et al [49] | 49 | GDM | 20 | 0 | 19 | ↓ pp with lispro |
| Masson [56] | 76 | T1DM | 76 | 0 | 0 | 6 SABs, 7 LGA, 4 CM, 6 laser therapy |
| Persson et al [57] | 33 | T1DM | 16 | 0 | 17 | ↓ A1C and pp with lispro, but ↑ retinopathy in both |
| Loukovaara et al [58] | 69 | | 36 | 0 | 33 | ↓ A1C and pp with lispro; nulliparity ↑ retinopathy |
| Wyatt et al [50] | 500 | T1DM | 500 | 0 | 0 | 27 CM with A1C >2 SD mean nl in 1st trimester |
| Garg et al [51] | 62 | T1DM | 62 | 0 | 0 | ↓ A1C with lispro; no change retinopathy or albumin 24% LGA, 2 CM |
| Carr et al [55] | 9 | T1DM | 9 | 0 | 0 | Premeal equal to postprandial injection |
| Cypryk et al [54] | 71 | T1DM | 25 | 46 | — | No difference |
| Pettitt et al [52] | 27 | GDM | 0 | 13 | 14 | ↓ pp with aspart |
| Hod et al [53] | 330 | T1DM | 0 | 125 | 125 | ↓ hypo- and hyperglycemia |
| Total = 12 | 1425 | 1150 T1DM 275 GDM | 795 | 59 | — | Improved outcome with lispro or aspart |

*Abbreviations:* A1C, glycosylated hemoglobin; CM, congenital malformations; LGA, large-for-gestational-age infant; pp, postprandial level; SABs, spontaneous abortions; T1DM, type 1 diabetes mellitus.

and insulin aspart are as safe and maybe more efficacious than short-acting regular insulin.

## Long-acting insulin analogues and their use during pregnancy

### Insulin glargine

Insulin glargine is a human insulin analogue with an activity that results in a constant concentration and time profile over 24 hours with no pronounced peak. Insulin glargine, approved for clinical use in 2000, is obtained by adding to the human molecule of insulin 2 molecules of arginine to the c-terminal of β chain and replacing aspartic acid with glycine in position A 21. These changes result in the shifting of isoelectric point from pH 5.4 to 6.7, with a reduction in insulin solubility when injected subcutaneously and in the capacity for dimerization these characteristics confer greater stability and duration of action. Insulin glargine begins its action approximately 90 minutes after subcutaneous injection, lasts approximately 24 hours, and is considered peakless compared with neutral protamine Hagedorn (NPH) insulin. In nonpregnant insulin-requiring diabetic subjects, insulin glargine administration produces better reduction in values of fasting and postprandial plasma glucose concentrations and a decrease in nocturnal hypoglycemia events [59–69].

Although the long-acting insulin analogues may provide a better basal glycemic profile than human NPH in insulin-requiring nonpregnant diabetic subjects [63–69], the literature is sparse on the safety and efficacy of these analogues in pregnancy [63–69]. Table 2 summarizes the eight articles to date that report the outcome of pregnancies complicated by insulin-requiring diabetes in which women were treated with glargine insulin at some point in pregnancy. Although there were no reported cases of malformations, the total sample of women exposed to glargine during pregnancy was too small to make a conclusion (23 total diabetic women treated: 14 type 1 diabetic women, and 9 gestational diabetic women). In addition, birth weight was not consistently mentioned and the total dose of insulin was not related to gestational week or maternal weight, and thus the treatment protocol is impossible to derive from these studies. In addition, glucose control was inconsistently measured, and thus the comparison of glycemia that can be achieved with the use of glargine compared with that of NPH or an insulin infusion pump delivering aspart or lispro during pregnancy also cannot be derived thus far from the literature.

### Detemir

Insulin detemir is another long-acting insulin analogue, pending US Food and Drug administration approval. The mechanisms of protracted action of insulin detemir include increased hexamer stability, binding to

Table 2
Use of long-acting insulin glargine in pregnancy

| Studies | Number of patients | Type of diabetes | Dose of glargine | Outcome |
|---|---|---|---|---|
| Woolderink et al [68] | 7 | T1DM 2: 1st and 2nd trimester 5: 1st, 2nd, and 3rd trimester | — | Delivered at 37–40 weeks; birth weight 4180 g (2,475–4,675 g) A1C 6.4% (5.2–8.1%) No CM |
| Graves et al [69] | 4 | GDM | 44 U mean (10–78 U) | 2 ↑ fasting glucose 1 LGA 1 daytime hypoglycemia No cases of nocturnal hypoglycemia |
| Dolci et al [67] | 1 | T1DM & Addison's Disease | 2nd trimester | Compared to NPH in 1st trimester better control with glargine |
| Di Cianni et al [63] | 5 | T1DM | 1st trimester | No CM |
| Devlin et al [61] | 1 | T1DM | 2nd and 3rd trimester | Better glycemia with glargine than NPH |
| Holstein et al [64] | 1 | T1DM | 1st, 2nd and 3rd trimester | Better glycemia with glargine than NPH |
| Torlone et al [66] | 6 | T1DM | 1st, 2nd, and 3rd trimester | Normal outcome |
| Carrona et al [65] | 1 | T1DM | 1st, 2nd, and 3rd trimester | 3540 g male infant |
| Total articles | Total treated with glargine | Type of diabetes | Dosage | Outcome |
| 8 | 21 | 14 T1DM 9 GDM | Average dose of glargine insulin 18–75 U/d | No congenital malformations but macrosomia rate is not possible to calculate from these reports |

*Abbreviations:* A1C, glycosylated hemoglobin level; CM, congenital malformations; LGA, large-for-gestational-age infant; pp, postprandial level; SABs, spontaneous abortions; T1DM, type 1 diabetes mellitus.

albumin at the subcutaneous injection site and in the circulation [70–72]. The benefits of insulin detemir, such as improved glycemic control, lowered within-subject variation, reduced nocturnal hypoglycemic events, and no weight gain has been shown in patients who have type 1 diabetes [73,74]. However, there are no clinical studies performed using insulin detemir in pregnant women who have diabetes. Animal reproduction studies in rabbits and rats have not revealed any differences between insulin detemir and human insulin regarding embryotoxicity and teratogenicity [75].

## Potential risks associated with insulin analogues

### Insulin and IGF-1 receptor binding affinity

There are hypothetical reasons to consider increased IGF-1 activity undesirable in pregnancy. During gestation, the female reproductive system undergoes dramatic changes to accommodate the development of the fetus. IGF-1 facilitates the implantation of the human embryo in the endometrium. Disturbance of IGF-1 functions could result in spontaneous miscarriage, preeclampsia, and defects of the embryo [76]. It is well known that the incidence of spontaneous miscarriage due to malformations of the fetuses during early pregnancies is much higher in women who have poorly controlled diabetes than in nondiabetic pregnancies. The mechanisms for the abortion and malformation are not completely understood. There are some factors that presumably play important roles in this process: inherited genetic abnormalities of the fetus, lack of endogenous insulin in maternal serum in type 1 diabetes, and embryotoxic effects of the diabetic serum [77,78]. Some researchers suspect that altered insulin and IGF-1 serum levels are candidates to account for dysregulation of trophoblast proliferation and invasion. In late pregnancy, the placenta produces a large amount of human placental growth hormone to regulate the flow of nutrients to the placenta to support fetal growth [79]. Like growth hormone, the effects of human placental growth hormone are mediated through IGF-1 and IGF-binding proteins. An insulin analogue that has high affinity for IGF-1 receptor might influence the natural processes mediated by IGF-1. Furthermore, increased human placental growth hormone and progesterone levels also account for increased insulin resistance and reduced insulin sensitivity during the last trimester.

The actions of insulin are mediated through binding of the insulin molecules to the insulin receptors located on the membrane of the target cells. IGF-1 receptor shares structural similarity to insulin receptor. IGF-1 can bind to the insulin receptor and insulin is capable of binding to the IGF-1 receptor. However, natural insulin binds to IGF-1 receptor with 1000-fold lower affinity than insulin binding to the insulin receptor, and insulin has a 1000-fold lower affinity than IGF-1 for the IGF-1 receptor [71]. The new insulin analogues all have modifications in their amino acid sequences or legitimate opportunities for self-advancement and characterized by low self-esteem, frustrated ambition and low expectations will manifest a code of behaviour which has at its centre values which differ from mainstream culture and which demonstrate hopelessness and nihilism. The crimes of car-theft, joy-riding, burglary and vandalism which characterize the rising crime practices in such localities are precisely the kind of crime that such commonsense assumptions might predict.

More scientific evidence of a link between unemployment and crime has been provided by a major study based at Cambridge University (Wells, 1994 & 1995). Wells suggests that the failure of Home Office research to recognize a link between unemployment and crime lies in its failure to recognize unemployment as a 'lagging' indicator of crime levels. Wells suggests that abundant evidence exists for a clear link between the business cycle and levels of property crime but that Home Office research fails to recognize that unemployment lags behind the business cycle and consequently blurs the statistical correlation. Wells concludes: 'The fact is the nation's unemployment black spots ..... are also its crime black spots.... The reason our great urban conurbations are the nation's crime spots reflects poor regional/national economic performance, particularly rapid de-industrialisation in recent years.'(1995, p6).

This evidence does much to dispel Government rhetoric about rising crime as a symptom of moral decline and inadequate punishment, and clearly lays the blame for the rising rates of property and car-crime at the door of unemployment and the failure of the New Right to see the securing of higher levels of employment as a legitimate and necessary concern of government.

There is an additional component of the New Right contribution to the rising rate of crime in working-class communities. The celebration of the enterprise culture and the influence of market-forces has penetrated deeply into young working-class consciousness. Whilst the traditional political collectivism of the working-class has often been exaggerated, the

17

generally collectivist value system of working-class communities is an established social fact (Bott 1971, Goldethorpe et al, 1968). Strong family and community networks, clear patterns of socialization in work and trade unions and the influence of peer behaviour have conventionally ensured that working-class behaviour is modified in the interests of significant others. This form of collectivism has been an important regulator of the excesses of behaviour in working-class communities and traditionally has ensured that crime is not generally committed against the home community. However, fifteen years of individualist ideology in a wide range of social contexts has done much to erode this intrinsic set of collectivist behaviour patterns. The demise of collectivized experience in work-place cultures such as mining, coupled with the decline of the corresponding political organizations of trade unions and popular Labour Party membership, have been a secondary feature of the decline of the traditional industries in South and North Wales.

Changes in the school curriculum and a wider influence of business people in school management have ensured the trickling down of enterprise and individualist values in school culture. Children participate in enterprise activities which teach business values which cut across the core value system of working-class communities. The New Right has achieved a strategy which propagandizes possessive individualism in the most pervasive manner. Additionally, the leisure patterns of working-class communities have become more individualized and the general emphasis on consumption in society has raised aspirations without raising incomes. The consequences are a ready acceptance on the part of working-class youth to lay claim to the benefits of the consumer society with little reflection on the methods by which the benefits are accrued.

ESRC-sponsored research by Dr John Beynon at the University of Glamorgan clearly indicates an entrepreneurial culture in the violent young men interviewed as part of a project on violent male culture in South Wales. Many offenders saw themselves as fulfilling the values of Thatcherism and saw no

18

contradiction in their use of violence as a means to achieving the valued goods of a consumer society. The politics of possessive individualism which have characterized Britain since 1979 have inevitably devalued the traditional collectivist ethos of working-class communities. The consequence is that the vast majority of property crime is experienced by the poor as a result of the actions of their neighbours and peers (Wells 1995). The young working-class male perpetrates the majority of his crimes against his own community.

Often linked with discussions of crime is the related issue of drug-abuse. One clear consequence of the excluded life-style of the working-class estates in Wales is the response in terms of drug-abuse as a palliative for the poor quality of life which such locations offer. Interviews with agencies in South Wales suggest significant changes to the pattern of drug use in the 1990s. Use of cannabis has escalated from unproblematic leisure use to habitual and routine use as a tranquillizer. Additionally, prescribed tranquillizers are traded freely and the use of amphetamines has grown considerably. Of greater concern is the increasing supply of cocaine, its derivatives, and heroine, often at prices which reflect local incomes. Again, these problems are clearly associated with key housing-estates in the region. Taff Ely Borough Council in Mid Glamorgan recognizes drug-related crime as the most serious problem on its housing-estates and now pursues a policy of eviction for convicted drug-dealers.

The discussion of poverty in this essay has in many ways been abstract. The statistics and social trends examined are one step away from the daily reality of poverty in Wales. Poverty has to be lived to fully understand its nature. The experience of poverty is varied and influenced primarily by the life-stages individuals move through. From deprived childhoods to cold and hungry old age, sections of the population in Wales will spend a lifetime in poverty. No statistics can measure the frustration, powerlessness and lost opportunities of such a waste of human resources. Discussions with agencies working with the poor in Wales paint a

19

depressing picture of a numbing life-style without hope or enjoyment.

That picture is of a constant struggle to make ends meet. Families with children exist on a daily income of as little as £2.50 after housing cost. The constant juggling of limited financial resources absorbs all the efforts of the waking day and saps energy. The burden of debt prevents forward planning and ensures that meagre incomes are substantially committed to clearing past expenditure whilst building new debts in the present. Once in this situation the poverty trap ensures that the poor pay more for almost every aspect of their consumption. Heating, food, clothing and transport all cost more when the individual is excluded by low income from the retail revolution which has swept Wales in the 1980s. Poor families are excluded from sources of credit and thrown into the hands of money-lenders who prey on the deprived estates in Wales. To live in poverty is to live in fear of eviction and repossession. It is to live with the threat and reality of disconnection of vital services such as water and electricity. It is to live in fear of the next knock on the door.

For the young living in poverty in Wales, the life is one without horizons and with limited ambitions. Trapped in communities without employment and with no social facilities, it is a life of drift and decline. Street-corners and empty houses offer gathering places where the inevitable companions are alcohol, drugs and solvents and a slide into petty-crime and delinquency. In a world without jobs other sources of identity and status come to the fore and are defined by the distorted values of the criminal sub-culture which inevitably emerges. Stealing and driving fast cars becomes a way of stating transition to manhood and maintaining a place in the local social hierarchy. Denied the transition to adulthood traditionally offered by work and marriage, young working-class males have established their own value-system which centres on violence and machismo and is now likely to permanently feature in the culture of the region.

Even now a return to full employment is unlikely to undo the damage of twenty years of economic decline.

The powerlessness experienced by the poor is overwhelming. The poor have virtually no arena where they can actively make decisions over the course of their lives. Income is committed before it is received and almost every aspect of their lives is determined by the officials who administer the benefit systems, the employment exchange, the training scheme and the local authority housing. The limited stability they experience can be jeopardized or lost by the decision of a bureaucrat in any of the departments they constantly have to negotiate with to secure their daily requirements. The rules of the benefit system effectively preclude education, training and voluntary work and individuals slip into a fatalism and passivity which compounds the hopelessness of their situation.

The effects on health of a life of poverty are incalculable. Physical health deteriorates early in the face of poor diet and reliance on cheap, high-fat sources of energy. Several studies have demonstrated that people in Britain today regularly experience hunger as a result of lack of money to buy food. Diseases of poverty and malnutrition are returning to the communities of Wales, exemplified by a noticeable increase in the incidence of tuberculosis. Alcohol and cigarette consumption are an inevitable by-product of the powerlessness and hopelessness of the life-style described by the agencies working with the poor communities. Tranquillizer dependence is endemic and little official attempt has been made to map the extent of illegal drug-use. The poor are excluded from life itself; they will die younger and experience poorer quality of life in the face of higher incidences of ill-health and incapacity. The levels of those registered permanently sick have risen constantly throughout the last decade.

One thing more than any other characterizes life for the poor in the 1990s in comparison to the past; the awareness of exclusion is highly developed in those who are excluded. The poor live in a society which is replete with the imagery of

21

affluence and wealth, and poverty in the 1990s is exaggerated by the inequality which has developed with it. The socially excluded are conscious and aware of the benefits of life in an affluent society which they are prevented from enjoying. The Rowntree Foundation Inquiry into Income and Wealth (1995) has left no doubt as to the increasing polarization of British society since 1977. Following a brief postwar period when income and wealth converged, the trend since 1977 is for the poor to become poorer and the remainder of society to become more affluent. The pervasive influence of the visual media has ensured that the poor are bombarded daily with knowledge of their poverty and exclusion, leaving them alienated and detached from a commitment to the society which excludes them.

This unemployment crisis has been demonstrated to trigger a more serious social crisis with a web of deprivation and exclusion. The high level of unemployment is tearing at the fabric of working-class communities in ways which have consequences for all of Welsh society. These communities have constituted the backbone of Welsh society in the nineteenth and twentieth centuries. They have added a cultural diversity which has ensured the survival of a Welsh identity which moves beyond the limited consideration of language and Cymric tradition which form the basis of the 'imagined community' (Anderson, 1983) of the Welsh middle-classes, the Welsh-speaking literati and intelligentsia. The dynamism of working-class culture has structured the politics and the culture of Wales and given it a radicalism and a world-wide reputation for community and mutual aid. It is these characteristics of our working-class communities which are being destroyed by the process of unemployment and social exclusion. In their place is left a weakened and struggling communalism and a highly atomized and individualized culture. The experience of poverty is an isolated one. Communal responses are few and far between and the fabric of communities is under great stress. We must act before that fabric is torn asunder.

## Towards the formation of a new politics

The solution to the crisis I have identified has to be a political solution. Wales has suffered acutely from the effects of fifteen years of New Right politics. A radical programme of political change is required to reverse those effects and to secure a new platform for the modernization and development of Welsh society. The scale of the problem to be tackled requires a radical rethink of the politics of the whole post-war period which have allowed the gradual return to the conditions which the 1945 Labour Settlement claimed to eradicate. British social democracy has failed the people of Wales and a new politics is required if there is to be any quality in the Welsh way of life in the new century.

The first requirement of any new basis for radicalism in Wales must be the realization that the process affecting the communities of Wales, even in the most rural enclaves, are the consequences of global events and practices. Wales cannot be seen as separate and distinct from the economic forces which create similar effects in Taiwan or the Basque region, Portugal or Arkansas. The villages of Wales are embedded in a world capitalist economy which shifts Japanese television production to Mid Glamorgan and imports coal through Cardiff docks from South Africa. We can afford no sense of independence from these processes and our political programmes must recognize and ameliorate their effects. We must be armed with an acute knowledge of the place of our nation within this global economic framework. Additionally, the politics of Wales are caught up in the global ideological struggles which have characterized world politics in the post-war period. Only through recognizing this global context and by working through its consequences can a new form of politics be found. The global issues must be addressed before the local difficulties can be resolved.

It is in this ideological arena that much of the struggle must take place. One of the major difficulties preventing the emergence of a new form of politics in Wales, and more generally on a global scale, is the ideological effects of the

23

collapse of the Soviet Union and its subject states. The revolutions which swept through Eastern Europe in the closing years of the 1980s have thoroughly redefined the political agenda in the western world. The collapse of the major ideological opponent of western liberal democracy has successfully removed key terms from the political vocabulary. Words such as socialism, equality and liberty have become identified with a failed and badly tainted social experiment. The worst excesses of the various Soviet-style regimes have been presented as a powerful demonstration of the intrinsic dangers contained within the philosophy of socialism as a doctrine. Western liberal democracies have engaged in a triumphalism about the end of struggle between socialism and capitalism. Events in Tianamen Square have highlighted the evil nature of the surviving communist regimes and any form of socialist project is deemed guilty by association. Claims have been made that western liberal democracy is now established as the final version of human consciousness and that it has established a permanent global consensus for the principles of the market-place. Francis Fukuyama (1989) exemplifies such claims in his perceptions about the 1989 revolutions signifying an end to the ideological struggles which have characterized history. For him Western democracy will be the final form of human government.

Not content with such a resounding victory over its long-standing ideological opponent, the triumphant victor stands astride its body and declares a war on history. Theories of post-modernism emerge to declare that the root of the evils of socialism are to be found in the Enlightenment project itself. For three hundred years we have mistakenly placed our faith in the power of human reason. A 'grand narrative' has been followed which bound us to unrealizable ideals which themselves have created human misery. It is claimed we have mistakenly thought that we understood the world and that we could, as a result, change it for the better. The knowledge we have of the world has been shown to be fallacious and the source of mistaken attempts to engineer social progress. Indeed, the concept of progress itself

24

has been challenged and set aside and parity claimed for all systems of thought. The attempt to promote socialism over capitalism is presented as a mistake of history which can only be redressed by accepting the chaos of the market-place and the struggle of everything against everything.

I shall not be concerned here to develop a critique of the excesses of post-modern epistemology. Its relativism and, at times, absurd reductionism are self-evident. However, I shall simply re-assert the belief that the world can be understood, that there is meaning to be derived and that it is possible to communicate and share that meaning. The result is an ability not simply to understand the world but to change it in ways we choose. However, the postmodern writers have forced us to recognize that the world is constantly changing and a 'truth' written over one hundred years ago is not necessarily true now. Similarly, theories which were meaningful in the early development of the industrial revolution are not necessarily of value today. The strategies of change we adopt must be informed by the past but they must be a product of the present, rooted in the social and economic conditions of our times. We must develop a progressive strategy which is possible to sustain and which does not appeal to a terminology and a doctrine which no longer reflect reality.

We must begin by challenging the ways in which the core doctrine of socialism has been ridiculed and de-legitimized as a strategy for the improvement of human existence. The principles of socialism are regarded as naive and utopian in the face of the reality of human existence which is perceived as inevitably 'nasty, brutal and short'. Claims of the existence of altruism and self-sacrifice are denied in the face of possessive individualism and the triumph of the market competitive ethic. How can a new politics, which places centrally the poor and the socially-excluded, emerge in such a hostile environment? How can those concerned with redressing gross inequality and the waste of human potential struggle against the apparent victory of a social system which produces poverty as one of its necessary by-products?

The starting-point has to be with issues of morality. Those who retain a sense that some of the features of the Enlightenment project remain valid objectives for a progressive society must begin to reclaim a sense of morality for those objectives. Those who feel that the existence of poverty can be objectively verified and that such an existence ridicules the claims to democracy made by liberal capitalist societies must reassert a critique of the morality of free enterprise capitalism. Those who feel that the international swings and roundabouts of the capitalist world economy exploit and discard whole nations at will must propagate a sense of outrage at the human misery left in the wake of wholesale movements of capitalist production.

It must be clearly demonstrated that liberal democracy fails in its own project of providing liberty and democracy for its citizens. The detailed practices of social exclusion given earlier in this essay demonstrate the failure of full active citizenship to be achieved by significant proportions of the population in Wales and in the other liberal democracies of Europe. Within the European Union, 50 million people are living in poverty (Williams, 1992). This invalidates any claim that liberal democracy might make to be the highest form of human government. It must be demonstrated that such liberal democracies fail in their ability to provide the welfare rights of employment, good housing, effective education and efficient health-care which must be seen as the most basic and fundamental rights in all societies. Without them the ability to participate as citizens in the practice of political and civil rights is meaningless. The ability of an illiterate to vote is the negation of political freedom and the meaningful participation of unemployed and poverty-stricken individuals in the benefits of contemporary society is impossible. The partial citizenship of all those affected by poverty and its consequences negate the very concept of democracy which is at the heart of the liberal democratic philosophy. The new politics must emphasize the right to participate and advance a programme for democracy with a real level of devolved responsibility to local decision-making

26

bodies. Political participation must once again become a right which is valued and an obligation which is fulfilled. To secure the reinsertion of political participation into popular culture requires the propagation of a view that participation produces results. It requires a reconnection of political participation with influence over decision-makers at both local and national level. The more power is devolved to local institutions the more likely such a culture is to re-emerge. Wales needs a new sense of freedom with which to motivate the excluded.

Unfortunately, the opposite has occurred. The ascendancy of the New Right has seen a return to the narrow economic freedoms of classical liberalism. The philosophies of Hayeck have triumphed over the philosophy of Beveridge. In Hayeck's view the state's acceptance of any responsibility for welfare provision signals the end of freedom as it inevitably ties the state to satisfying the insatiable demands of society for such provision. Thus begins a slide towards totalitarianism as the state develops the necessary planning mechanisms to organize the welfare state and negates freedom through its taxation of economic activity (Hayeck, 1944). The only freedoms guaranteed in the contemporary philosophy of the market-place are the freedom to accumulate wealth and to retain it without state interference. This has been demonstrated most clearly in the controversy over salaries for the heads of the newly privatized public utilities. One of the most offensive examples has been evident here in Wales with the vast salary increases of Welsh Water/Dwr Cymru's Chief Executive. Such is the public outrage over such issues that the normally conservative *South Wales Echo* has run a campaign which contrasts his increasing wealth with the plight of those suffering automatic disconnection of water-supply by the deployment of smart-card water-meters. The *Echo* has also printed a regular update of the value of SWALEC Chairman Wynford Evans's share option package. The 'freedom' of the New Right is experienced by a tiny minority.

Unregulated behaviour in the City and Britain's financial institutions has also tarnished the image of the free market, free-

27

for-all but without apparent effect on the dogma of a Government which sees intervention as politically unacceptable. The argument that these activities will create the wealth which 'trickles down' to improve the lives of the poor has been demonstrated to be false. In Britain, fifteen years of privatization and unregulated financial speculation have failed to create a share-owning democracy or any hint of improved incomes for the poor. In fact the opposite has occurred: 'In the last decade, the living standards of the poor and affluent marched in opposite directions. For the first time in recent years, there is official evidence that the real disposable incomes of the poorest actually fell. Between 1979 and 1988/9, the poorest tenth of the population saw their real income (after housing costs) fall by 6%; the average rose by 30%, while the richest tenth enjoyed a staggering rise of 46%'. (Oppenheim, 1993, p.1, quoting DSS sources)

The regional concentration of these financial activities has ensured that no benefits have been experienced in any of the peripheries of Great Britain and Wales has certainly seen no advantage from the 'financial revolution' of the 1980s. Indeed the privileging of the City interest in government policies throughout the 1980s severely damaged manufacturing capitalism in Britain and directly contributed to the collapse of employment in manufacturing in Wales which occurred in that decade. The most damaging of the policies was the maintenance of artificially high rates of interest in the quest to maintain deflationary pressure in the economy. The result was an eventual collapse of consumer demand and a punishing debt burden for small businesses.

The failure of liberal democracy is also its failure to create any climate in which social justice can be established. The liberal democratic conception of social justice requires society's members to be rewarded on the basis of merit. The creation of a meritocracy has been at the heart of social democratic politics in Britain since the end of the second world war. Major educational reforms, the advances of the welfare state until the early 1970s and the pursuit of full employment within the Keynesian

28

strategies of the post-war consensus, have all failed to establish the context of equal opportunities which a meritocracy requires. The fundamentally most significant determinant of an individual's outcome in life is their social class of origin. Studies from Glass (1954) to Goldthorpe (1980) have demonstrated that real vertical movement in British society remains difficult, with the division between manual and mental labour representing the most significant barrier to social mobility. The new politics must declare the meritocratic dream dead and build a more radical vision of social justice which has a sense of equality as its founding principle.

Socialist conceptions of social justice seek to combine criteria of need, equality and merit. Few socialists would advocate the creation of a society with absolute equality as its objective. However, there must be equality of need to ensure that every individual has his or her basic needs satisfied. Equality of housing, education and health-care is a prerequisite of a society in which the social exclusion and poverty discussed in this essay is abolished. Having established a basic standard of living for all, a society can create a number of criteria for establishing the distribution of additional rewards with the merit of the individual's contribution to society as the most likely qualification. There will be a requirement to limit the differential of rewards in such a society to ensure that the social system remains acceptable to all participants. In contrast to a system of social justice based on these criteria, the current philosophy of the New Right is easy to ridicule and oppose. Its claims that it preserves natural inequalities and reflects the diverse distribution of human talents has created the most unequal distribution of benefits in society since the Victorian era. The beneficiaries of the inequality are highly visible and the public is outraged at the lack of control over private wealth. Surprisingly, no one voices an alternative sense of social justice.

Strategies in the quest for the new politics must be learned from the New Right itself. Stuart Hall (Hall & Jacques, 1983) drew attention to the ways in which the Thatcherite project to

29

create a new hegemony in British politics sought to align itself with public concerns about British society and the welfare state which were evident at the beginning of the 1980s. In a process of 'resonance' Thatcherism took those public concerns and restated them in exaggerated form and played them back to the public in an amplified reworking of the original ideas. This was especially evident around issues of rising crime and social security 'scrounging'. By deploying this strategy the Thatcher governments were able to wean the British people away from the politics of welfarism to a suspicion of the ability of the state to offer welfare support and a distaste for those who are dependent on it .

A similar strategy of resonance must be adopted in the quest for a new radical politics in Wales. Despite the major successes of Thatcherism in shifting the political ground to the right, it failed to rewrite totally the post-war settlement of the Labour years and the British public remain attached to a strong sense of communal responsibility and distrust of market forces in the contexts of health, education and housing. It is this distrust which the new politics must pick up, amplify and play back to a public which is naturally sympathetic to a critique of market forces. All classes now share a distrust and distaste for the marketization of public utilities and the public services. The new politics must address these concerns about the excesses of the application of market principles, rework them and replay them as a critique of the concept of the market itself. This is precisely the strategy adopted by the New Right in its programme of action against the welfare state. In Wales we are in a position to lead such a campaign. The New Right has never enjoyed legitimacy in Wales. The unique configuration of social forces in Wales has forced the Welsh Office to continue with interventionist strategies whilst central government moved further towards a minimalist state. The political culture in Wales has imposed a different strategy on the successive occupants of the Welsh Office and has constantly rejected the philosophy of the market-place. Unfortunately, the political opposition has done nothing to focus that dissent and give it voice. This is the task for the new politics.

Additionally, the new politics must be a popular movement in that it must resonate with popular concerns and lead popular opinion. Hall & Jacques (1983) saw one of the key features of Thatcherism as its appeal to populist trends in the political culture. Of key importance was its emphasis on authoritarianism and its successful linkage between crime, declining morality and the permissive society. This enabled an increasingly authoritarian strategy to be adopted which has culminated in the Criminal Justice Act which attempts to make alternative lifestyles and beliefs systems illegal. One of Italian Marxist Antonio Gramsci's great insights was to see that working-class consciousness has an alarming capacity to contain quite contradictory elements including fascism, liberalism, and socialism. The new politics must create a populism which feeds the socialist and collectivist components of consciousness to create a new moral system which foregrounds traditional concerns with the welfare of others. This is an important strand of Welsh culture which has not been eliminated by the New Right. However, it has been weakened and needs urgent sustenance which must come from a political movement which offers confirmation of the value and desirability of a society in which these values are celebrated.

One entry point available to the new politics into such a populist programme is through the concept of community. All political parties have appealed to the sense of community and it surfaces repeatedly in sociological studies as one of the primary sources of identity for individuals. The New Right has robbed us of a developed sense of community and reduced us to individual or family-based consumers. Where it employs the concept of community it has reduced it to an image of fortress communities under siege from the criminal and delinquent products of the permissive years. The new politics must reclaim a socialist sense of community which transcends social divisions and creates a sense of shared responsibility for all members of the community. The fear of crime must be replaced with a clear focus on the causes of crime which are, in reality, external to our communities. Unemployment and poverty can be demonstrated

31

to be an external threat to our communities which can be opposed politically. We must diffuse the blame we place on the poor and replace it with a vivid sense of the real cause of crime. We must identify the part played by the poverty and alienation which affects those who have never worked and who subsequently lose their respect and commitment for the communities in which they live.

Finally, we must learn from the New Right that the language of politics is important. The skill of Mrs Thatcher was to use a populist vocabulary which translated complex political issues to issues of emotional appeal and created prejudice against traditional collectivist values in the community. The language of the new politics must seek to reverse this. A new rhetoric of socialism must be developed which avoids the terminology and strategy of the post-war period which is now cast into ill-repute by the New Right denigration of its purpose. We must find a new language with which to promote the core values of socialism. One potential avenue for this lies in the concept of citizenship. The ability to participate fully in society is one of the central principles of liberal democracy. If it is failing in this, as it so clearly is, it is a failed political and economic system. The sense of that failure is everywhere. In the dole-queues and the rising crime-statistics, in the urban poverty and the failure of the economy, we see its failure. The public is aware of the failure but are bombarded with messages that all is well and that the system works. Non-participation and exclusion are presented as the consequence of some personal failing. We must stress that the failure is of a political and social system and not a failure of individuals. The advantages of citizenship must be spelt out to those sections of the population who have given up on their participation and who no longer claim the right to participate. More importantly, we must raise the ability to recognize the right to participate in a generation which is growing up in a climate of social-exclusion. That generation lives in a culture which does not inform it of its rights as citizens and creates an experience which stresses the futility of attempting to participate as such.

The final component of a strategy based on the concept of citizenship requires us to consider the nature of the political unit we claim citizenship of.

One of the key components of the programme which must be adopted by any radical movement in Wales is the achievement of independence from the British state. The motivation for this claim is not only to recognize the cultural diversity of Wales but to contribute to the demise of the British Union. The existence of a United Kingdom of Great Britain is a legacy of the development of the greatest imperial power in history. The society created by the political and economic development of the British Empire is intrinsically conservative and reactionary. Indelibly stamped with militarism and monarchism, it is a society within which hierarchy and inequality are celebrated as part of the national culture. The British class-system continues to be replicated in an educational system which has the private schools on the one hand and under-funded, overcrowded comprehensives on the other. No reform of such an intrinsically divided society is possible. Fifty years of a comprehensive welfare state have failed to scratch the surface of inequalities of rank and privilege which characterize British society. The Celtic fringe has fared no better. Any claims that Scotland and Wales are more egalitarian societies are absurd. The myth of the classless *gwerin* in Welsh nationalist ideology must be dispelled by a full awareness of the divisions within Wales and their close relationship to the patterns of patronage and status operated by the British state. Breakaway from the British state is advocated because of its weakening of the power of the British state. As a consequence, all forms of devolution of power are to be supported but only as a basis for the radical transformation of the political system in which Wales exists. The erosion of the British state will permit an increasing influence from Europe where the social democratic tradition has fared a little better than in Britain during the years of the New Right and a strong socialist lobby still survives.

And now we arrive at the most difficult questions of all. Where in Welsh politics can we look to discover the source of this new radicalism which is so urgently needed? Where can we discover the moral outrage which will give it its energy? Where can we find the political will to engage in a struggle which stands against the tide of history?

## Wales and the new politics

How can the new politics emerge in a Wales which has been so debilitated by the economic shifts of the global market and which has preserved itself very much in the style of the failed politics of social democracy? Can we expect a people which has been weakened by economic collapse and dispirited by fifteen years of effective disenfranchisement within an elective dictatorship to develop a new radical politics? History suggests we might. Welsh political culture is distinguished by a tradition of radicalism. That radicalism has been expressed in a variety of forms, shaped by the specific circumstances of a different era. The history of Welsh socio-political movements and events are a testimony to the influence of a comparatively small nation on the development of radicalism in Europe. The Daughters of Rebecca, the Scotch Cattle, the Merthyr Rising, the Chartists, Nonconformism, Welsh Liberalism, the South Wales Miners' Federation, the Independent Labour Party, The Labour Party, Plaid Cymru, Cymdeithas yr Iaith Gymraeg all clearly demonstrate the willingness of people in Wales to form or link to progressive social movements which swim against the political tide of their times. There is a heritage and a culture of radicalism in Wales which can be revived in the face of the scale of problems now affecting Welsh communities.

The kind of radicalism which dressed the Daughters of Rebecca or marched Chartists to Newport we can expect to have disappeared. It was the product of the maelstrom of social change in a Wales hurtling into the industrial age. The dislocation of centuries of custom and practice inevitably threw into existence a politics of violent and chaotic protest. We have no right to mourn the departure of that kind of radicalism as the social conditions which brought it into existence have matured into other less

34

evident forms of poverty and inequality. However, there is another form of radicalism which we might have expected to survive the march of Wales from industrialism to post-industrialism. The communities which coal and metal production gave birth to still exist. They are again characterized by unemployment and poverty to an extent which set a thousand feet out on the hunger-marches of the 1930s. The social conditions in our industrial towns and villages are some of the worst in Europe and the population beset by poor housing, ill health and poor education. We have a right to expect the Labour Party in Wales to be leading the reaction against this situation. But the response to this Welsh situation is a silence. A silence which drapes the Welsh Labour Party with a shroud of inaction, a silence in which the only faint sound is the rattle of mayoral chains and the polite acceptance of seats in the Lords and other forms of Tory patronage. The Welsh Labour Party takes its inspiration and its orders from Westminster. Since the second World War it has sacrificed any sense of Welsh identity and worked within the British nationalism of the British Labour Party. To understand the failure of the Labour Party in Wales we have to initially place it in this wider British context.

The first issue to establish is that the British Labour Party is itself a failure. The Labour Party in Wales is part of a fifty-year project which has failed the working-class of Scotland, England, Ireland and Wales. This failure runs much deeper than its failure to secure election for nearly sixteen years. It is a failure which pre-dates the embarrassing débâcles of the '80s and '90s. It is a failure which begins in 1945 and marks a continued failure of the British Labour movement to radically challenge the basis of capitalism. The period 1945-1953 is frequently seen as the high point of British socialism and its establishment of a social democratic welfare state. Clearly, the reforms of the period represented huge advances for the working-class of Britain. Acute poverty was gradually eradicated and the '50s and '60s can be seen as a 'golden age' of welfare protection from the excesses of capitalist economic fluctuations. However, the whole period can be seen now as a series of compromises with capitalism which allowed its continued functioning in the conditions of the world economy in the aftermath of the second world war.

Rather than a programme of radical change, the reforms of 1945 and after can be seen as a continuance of the command economy of the war period itself. Rather than a radical challenge to capitalism, the Labour settlement can be seen as creating the conditions for the continued accumulation of capital. The reforms of the period created a new basis for hegemony which recognized and incorporated the changed aspirations of the working-class which had been raised by their struggle against fascism and the associated implicit promise of their own freedom when the war was won. The apparent radicalism of the period is riven with compromises which have constituted key fracture-lines for the welfare system in the period of challenge it has faced since the late 1960s. Compromises over private education, private medicine and over the extent and nature of social ownership ensured that the welfare state had a flawed foundation which revealed itself in the ease with which the New Right have managed to roll back welfare provision.

It should not be forgotten that the twin strategies of post-war economic and social policy were the work of Beveridge and Keynes, two Liberal thinkers. The Labour vision was dominated not by the socialist ethics of the labour movement but by the reformism of the Liberal intelligentsia. At that point in history the Labour Party divorced itself from its social origins and began an ever-widening division between the Party and its grass-roots support which has culminated in the recent rewriting of Clause IV. Never again has it directly represented the interests of the working people of Great Britain but has suffered the contradictory role of attempting to ameliorate the effects of capitalism whilst creating the conditions for its advancement.

The consequences of this basic failure are enormous and are reflected in every policy failure which has beset the Labour Party in office. It renders its social ownership strategy ineffective, it creates contradictions in its taxation policy. It renders the management of the economy senseless as it attempts to serve competing objectives and it ties foreign policy continually to an essential partnership with US capital. Little wonder that every Labour Party administration in the post-war period has failed to advance beyond the welfarism of 1945. It also ensured that in the first economic crisis to face the welfare mixed economy the Labour Party presided over sustained attacks on the living standards of the British people in a disastrous attempt to sustain the 1945 dream. The post-war settlement was not socialist; it continued a sustained strategy for the management of British capitalism. It was readily accepted by the Conservative Party and ensured the survival of the class-system and British militarism. It can certainly be accepted that the commitments to full employment and the creation and expansion of a welfare state were major elements in the post-war settlement. But these co-existed with support for the international reserve and transaction roles of sterling and for a military establishment and defence task which were incompatible with an effective KWS (Keynesian Welfare State)......this reveals the hybrid and contradictory character of the postwar settlement and the limits of social democratic hegemony therein'. (Jessop et al, 1988,p. 75)

What of the Welsh Labour Party? In Wales, Labour has compounded this failure of the Labour Party to represent its natural constituency. Episodes of corruption have punctuated a permanent complacency founded on unassailable majorities. Domination of constituency politics has been matched by a strangle-hold on local authorities which has only recently been challenged in South Wales by some Plaid Cymru successes in the Labour heartlands. The security of tenure of the town halls enjoyed by the Labour Party has created a conservative and reactionary political culture which has presided over the decline of our working-class communities. Slavish acceptance of central government spending cuts and an inability to lead and to focus massive public concern over issues such as housing and education, demonstrates that the Labour Party in Wales is ideologically bankrupt and undeserving of the continued faith the majority of

37

Welsh people place in it. Effectively, the radicalism of the working-class communities has run out into diluted streams of a crude municipalism with its own structure of rank and privilege.

Finally, to this British and Welsh failure of the Labour Party we must add the major rightward shift which dominates the Labour Party of the present time. It has accepted the definition of the political terrain provided by Thatcherism and has spent the last ten years divesting itself of the few remaining radical elements of its agenda. This process has recently focused on the issue of reform of Clause IV which has come to represent the struggle between the small Left rump of the Party and the right-wing politics of New Labour. In our quest for a source of the new politics in Wales we must turn away from a Party which removes its beliefs in social ownership at the time when all sections of the public are most disillusioned with the politics of privatization. At no time in the last fifteen years has the electorate been more receptive to arguments for the public ownership of the major utilities. The quest for the support of the English middle-classes will ensure that the Labour Party will be unable to serve the interests of the poor in Wales or, for that matter, anywhere else.

If we are forced to reject the Labour Party as a candidate for the role of leading the new politics in Wales, where else might we look? The nationalist movement is the only other candidate. The movement represents the other strand of radicalism in Welsh history. Motivated by very different concerns from those of the Labour Party, Welsh Nationalists have demonstrated a greater willingness to pursue their objectives by radical strategies. From the burning of the Penyberth bombing-school in 1936 to the campaigns of Cymdeithas yr Iaith Gymraeg (The Welsh Language Society) nationalists have frequently employed extra-parliamentary forms of political activity to considerable effect. However, the adoption of a parliamentary strategy by Plaid Cymru has effectively divided the nationalist movement into two strands . I shall look at each of these in turn.

The first is the linguistic and cultural movement in Wales. Exemplified by Cymdeithas yr Iaith Gymraeg, this movement has continued the early concern of Plaid Cymru with linguistic and cultural survival. It is this wing of the nationalist movement which has most readily employed non-violent direct action as a device for gaining publicity and for pressing its claims against authorities in Wales. In social origin, the movement has been largely middle-class and drawn from the Welsh-speaking areas of Wales. The language activists have been characterized by their youth and there is a strong connection between the movement and the Colleges of the University of Wales at Bangor and Aberystwyth. The movement has been extremely successful in pressing its demands and gaining concessions, especially from the Welsh Office and the language has a stronger base than any of the other Celtic languages.

Despite its radical strategies, the ideology of this movement has been far from radical. At its centre is a narrow cultural romanticism which is founded on a sense of linguistic élitism and exclusion. The Welsh-speaking middle-classes have managed to hegemonize definitions of Welshness to exclude the English-speaking culture of the industrial regions of Wales and have persuaded the English-speaking Welsh of their inferiority, founded on their failure to retain the mother-tongue. The Welsh-speaking community has engineered a social division in Wales based on a sense of high and low culture in which English-speakers are defined as not-Welsh. Driven by guilt and inferiority, the English-speaking working-class of Wales flock to send their children for education in a linguistic medium which has no connection with their social world. Already disadvantaged in the education system by the dynamics of their class, the children suffer the additional disadvantage of being educated in a medium which they will never speak at home and which they will forget within three years of leaving school. A chasm exists between working-class parents and school culture in general; when it is widened by the barrier of language, the effects on the educational attainment of working-class children is catastrophic. The Welsh-speaking middle-classes have perpetrated a desperate con-trick to underwrite the survival of their language.

There has been no attempt to link the survival of the language to the economic and social vitality of the society in which it has a rightful place. Language is seen as an end in itself, with no location of the strategy for linguistic survival in a vibrant economy and society. Declarations of its socialist intent by the language movement are meaningless and the structure of the political system of Wales is of secondary importance. The Conservative administrations of the Welsh Office have recognized the importance of language concessions in defusing discontent in Wales far more readily than the Labour Party ever did and the major concessions to the demands of the vociferous linguistic minority throughout the 1980s have ensured that a potentially radical element of Welsh society has been appeased. In the meantime the poor of Wales have descended deeper into their poverty.

Finally, in our quest for a radical leadership for the new politics we come to Plaid Cymru. On the face of it we are with a strong candidate. The Party seeks independence from the British State and a relocation of Wales within Europe. This was seen earlier as an essential component of any new politics which seeks to challenge the integrity of the British state and the inequalities of class and region it maintains. Most importantly the Party has made a clear declaration of its socialist principles and its concern to organize society around a decentralist emphasis on community. Both these strategies were identified earlier as important to the formation of a new politics in Wales. Does Plaid Cymru with its articulation of a politics of socialism and community offer us the source of a radical new politics?

To answer this question we must analyze the role performed by these concepts of socialism and community within the internal structure of the Party. Plaid Cymru has historically been divided between a concern for language and culture and a concern for economic development and progress. This division has never fitted easily within a rural/urban division and there is no suggestion here that this represents a geographical division between North and South. Rather, this dichotomy represents an ideological division within the Party which we can term culturalism and modernism. Since the 1960s modernism has prevailed and the defence of language and culture has been largely left to the language movement. Despite having its primary electoral base in Gwynedd the Party has pursued a strategy which has sought increased support in the heavy industrial communities, particularly in South Wales. The culturalist elements of the Party have been able to accept this and the socialist strategy it necessitates by responding to a specific ideological appeal to their sense of community. The term community has operated as a form of social cement which has bound the disparate elements of the Party together in the 1970s and 1980s.

The concept of community employed by Plaid Cymru has never been defined and it has retained an open meaning which allows individuals to insert their own sense of community into party rhetoric. Two dominant conceptions of community have existed. The first is a sense of rural community with an emphasis on kinship, neighbourhood and identifiable patterns of language, culture and religion. The second is a sense of industrial community associated with coal and steel production, with networks of mutual aid, traditions of working-class politics and labourism. As long as the meaning of the term community was not defined, all sections of the Party could feel loyalty to a concept of decentralist socialism founded in communities. Individuals could simply insert their own commonsense meaning for the term community, derived from their particular experience of life in Wales. A farmer on the Llŷn peninsula could feel as committed to the concept as a miner from Maerdy. The concept acted as an ideological and social cement which bound the Party together and allowed the project of the modernists to proceed.

Unfortunately, in the late 1980s a solvent appeared which rapidly dissolved this ideological cement and fractured the Party along traditional fault-lines. The solvent was in the form of a perceived crisis of inward migration and its effects on the rural communities of the Welsh-speaking heartlands. Suddenly, there was a perception of threat to the very communities with which significant proportions of the Party identified. A growing awareness emerged that the modernist leadership did not necessarily share the conception of community now coming to the centre of grassroots party concerns. The symbolism of community could no longer bind the Party together and the crisis emerged as a flurry of criticism of Party chairperson Dafydd Elis Thomas. This crisis effectively revealed that the deployment of the concepts of socialism and community within the Party had never been more than an ideological device which bound it together. Community and socialism have never been carefully defined by the Party and consequently have not been built into the programme of policies it pursues. However, the concepts have been more significant than mere political rhetoric. They have been the motivating principles for many of Plaid Cymru's members, but they have not formed a coherent policy base which members can rally to. Rather, they have remained open concepts to be interpreted at will by individual members and a coherent decentralist, socialist strategy has not emerged. It is this failing which demonstrates the inability of the Party to make gains in the industrial south during the 1980s. The community socialist basis is not visible outside the Party; it has existed only as an internal mechanism of party unity.

The conclusion has to be that Plaid Cymru is riven by a contradictory need to serve both its culturalist wing and its modernist wing. This contradiction at the heart of the Party makes it impossible for it to develop a fully radical programme which could protect the communities which are the concern of this essay. The poverty and social exclusion of the industrial areas can never be fully reconciled with the needs of the rural communities, although the levels of poverty may at times coincide. The different cultural basis of the politics of these different communities makes it impossible to develop a political programme of change which serves both.

The depressing conclusion is that neither the Labour Party in

Wales nor the nationalist movement can provide the new politics required from within their present structure and programmes. Significant contradictions within both political movements render it impossible for either to step into the political vacuum experienced by the excluded and the disenfranchized poor. Both parties are wedded to strategies which limit their potential to develop a radical alternative to the pursuit of social democracy via the parliamentary process. At this stage we can begin to draw a distinction between the party mechanisms and the individual members. It is very clear that there is a growing concern in Wales for our future direction of development and an emerging popular critique of the excesses of the market economy. Assisted by a burgeoning voluntary sector which is becoming increasingly politicized, there is a rising tide of dissent which no current political organizations are giving lead to. History demonstrates that such times are likely to produce new social movements to articulate these concerns. Should this occur there are legions of discontented members and supporters of both Labour and Plaid Cymru who would constitute a natural constituency for such a movement. Additionally, there are the poor themselves who, contrary to opinion, do not simply wait passively on the sidelines of society. They are organized into credit unions, tenants' associations and self-help and community groups of all kinds. Finally, there are the articulate middle-classes who—contrary to contemporary belief—are highly capable of support for radical causes. There is a growing distaste for the kind of society we have become. Many look to the United States as a mirror of the future and wish to avoid the destination we appear to be moving towards. No one wishes to live in a society characterized by no-go areas, infringement of our ability to relax in our own communities and surrounded by fear and concern for our children. There is a constituency awaiting a radical alternative which identifies the real causes of these trends and proposes significant means of reversing them.

The requirement is for a catalyst which brings these social forces together. The most likely candidate for the role is the next

General Election. The politics of Wales remains, for the moment, bound up with the politics of Britain. An election of another Conservative Government will provide a substantial impetus for the appearance of a radicalism, especially in the Celtic fringe which has so consistently rejected such governments in the past. Equally likely is that the election of a Labour Government which is itself a pale reflection of Conservatism may spark off the same process, although a time-lag may be an additional factor. The only other likely source of inspiration is from Europe and the comparisons we as a society make with our European counterparts. Increasingly, Britain appears isolated and antiquated. Our politicians reject the levels of social provision widely accepted as the norm in Europe and we endure wages which are a fraction of European workers. We shall eventually develop an awareness of the way in which the British State stands between us and social progress of a kind accepted as inevitable in the 1960s but which has since receded to a distant memory for the population of Britain. Finally, there is a spirit abroad in the world which challenges the historical pattern of domination, located in the nation state. Small nations are claiming their right to self-determination and see themselves better served by belonging to a decentralized and federal European Union. The British State may find itself unable to sustain its grip on Scotland and Wales.

For the people who live in deprivation and suffer social exclusion the task is urgent. No one speaks for them and their own voice is ignored. More and more individuals and communities face continued decline and decay as the erosion of the welfare safety-net proceeds apace. Children are being born in Wales today into a world which will cripple their physical, intellectual and emotional development. We can no longer stand by and blame them for it.

posttranslational modifications, such as acylation of the insulin molecules in the case of insulin detemir [80]. Such structural modifications sometimes lead to enhanced or reduced affinity for the insulin receptor and IGF-1 receptor. It has been reported that an insulin analogue B10Asp with a single amino acid substitution of aspartic acid for histidine for residue 10 of the β chain resulted in an increase in insulin and IGF-1 receptor affinity and demonstrated increased tumorigenic potential in female Sprague-Dawley rats [81].

Kurtzhals and colleagues [82] compared the metabolic and mitogenic potencies of several insulin analogues including B10Asp, insulin aspart, insulin lispro, insulin glargine, and insulin detemir to that of regular human insulin, and attempted to establish a correlation between the receptor binding affinity (to insulin receptor and IGF-1 receptor) and the metabolic and mitogenic potencies of these insulin analogues. They found that metabolic potency of insulin analogues correlated well with insulin receptor affinity, whereas mitogenic potency was generally more correlated with IGF-1 receptor affinity than with insulin receptor off-rates. It was reported that insulin glargine had a 6-fold increase in IGF-1 receptor affinity, and a corresponding 7-fold increase in mitogenic potency as measured in a human osteosarcoma cell line (Saos/B10) that has abundant IGF-1 receptors. The B10Asp analogue had a 9- to 10-fold increase in mitogenic potency, whereas insulin aspart, insulin lispro, and insulin detemir all had similar or reduced mitogenic potencies compared with human insulin [83]. However, some other studies using different cell lines have shown different results. A study using H9c2 cardiac myoblasts (which lack insulin receptor) showed that B10Asp had significantly higher affinity for IGF-1 receptor and greater mitogenic effects on these cells, whereas insulin glargine and native insulin were essentially equipotent [77]. In another study using differentiated cultured human skeletal cells from nondiabetic and diabetic subjects, Ciaraldi and colleagues [83] reported that human insulin and insulin glargine had similar mitogenic effects as determined by thymidine uptake into DNA, and the sensitivities and potencies were greatly reduced compared with IGF-1 ($<1\%$ of IGF-1). These researchers concluded that in a cell system representative of the relative insulin and IGF-1 receptor expression in human skeletal muscle cells, insulin glargine and native human insulin are comparable in receptor binding and metabolic responses, and that glargine does not display augmented mitogenic effects.

The IGF-1 signaling pathway is involved in different stages of pregnancy, and pregnancy is sensitive to alterations in the levels of these growth regulation hormones. Therefore, it may be desirable for a clinician to choose an insulin or insulin analogue with minimum IGF-1 activity while treating pregnant women who have diabetes. An example in recent development, insulin detemir, has a reduced affinity for IGF-1 receptor (approximately 1/10 that of human insulin) [83], which could be beneficial if pregnant women are susceptible to overstimulation of IGF-1 receptors. However, there are no data currently available on the use of insulin detemir during pregnancy.

The efficacy and safety of this new insulin analogue will need to be further assessed in pregnant women who have diabetes.

## Development of retinopathy during pregnancy

Many patients who have type 1 or type 2 diabetes suffer from microvascular complications such as retinopathy and nephropathy. The Diabetes Control and Complication Trial research group [77] reported that pregnancy was associated with an increase in the rate of retinopathy compared with nonpregnant women. The risk of worsening of retinopathy during pregnancy was 1.63 fold greater in the intensive treatment group, and was 2.5 fold greater in the conventional group than in a nonpregnant group. Furthermore, pregnancy is often associated with worsening of glycemic control, which is another contributing factor to the worsening of retinopathy [84–94]. The risk factors associated with progression of retinopathy during pregnancy include duration of diabetes, severity of retinopathy at conception, metabolic control, and coexisting hypertension. Results from many studies have indicated that rapid improvement in glycemic control was associated with progression of retinopathy in pregnant women as well as in nonpregnant patients who have diabetes. More recently, it has been suggested that insulin and IGF-1 may play a role in the development and progression of retinopathy. In an oxygen-induced mouse retinopathy model, knockout of insulin and IGF-1 receptors on vascular endothelial cells protected the animals from developing retinal neovascularization and showed a reduction of vascular mediators, such as VEGF, eNOS, and endothelin-1, with the effect of insulin being most significant [91].

There has been a case report that three pregnant women who had no detected background retinopathy developed bilateral proliferative diabetic retinopathy during their pregnancies while treated with insulin lispro [92]. It could not be determined whether the development of proliferative diabetic retinopathy was due to rapid tightening of glycemic control or due to the effects of insulin lispro, but it may be desirable to exercise caution if lispro is used during pregnancy in women who have a high risk of developing retinopathy [94]. No definite conclusions can be drawn until well-designed clinical trials are conducted to answer these questions.

## Summary

Depending on the type, severity, and stage of diabetes, patients may have only elevated postprandial glucose levels and normal fasting blood glucose levels, or the fasting glucose levels may be elevated as well. If postprandial glucose is the target of treatment, the rapid-acting insulin lispro and insulin aspart seem to be as safe and effective as regular human insulin in women who have GDM and achieve better postprandial glucose concentrations with less late postprandial hypoglycemia. If the patient has elevated fasting and postprandial blood glucose levels, and requires multiple daily injections to achieve good glycemic control, a basal-bolus regimen should be considered. The long-acting insulin analogues do not have as pronounced peak effect as NPH insulin and therefore cause less nocturnal hypoglycemia. The safety of these insulin analogues needs to be further established in pregnant women. Issues that will need to be further clarified include the question of whether these insulin analogues have teratogenic effects on the developing fetus, alter the balance between the binding affinity to IGF-1 receptor and insulin receptor, are associated with increased risk of retinopathy, or show increased antibody levels. Due to the lack of information in animal studies and high risk of clinical trials, it is unrealistic to expect results from large-scale, controlled clinical trials for evaluation of the safety profiles of these insulin analogues. For the time being, clinicians will have to rely on their knowledge of the pharmacology of the treatments, sporadic case reports, and their own judgment when making decisions regarding whether or not an insulin analogue should be used in pregnant women who have diabetes. Future research must also include the development of insulins that perfectly match physiologic insulin profiles during pregnancy. Although portal insulin delivery and inhaled insulin delivery have been associated with a closer match to endogenous insulin secretory profiles than subcutaneously injected insulin, the safety and efficacy of these routes of insulin delivery for pregnant women also need to be studied.

# References

[1] Pedersen J. Course of diabetes during pregnancy. Acta Endocrinol (Copenh) 1952;9:342–7.
[2] Mills JL, Knopp RH, Simpson JL, et al. Lack of relation of increased malformation rates in infants of diabetic mothers to glycemic control during organogenesis. N Engl J Med 1988; 318:671–6.
[3] Mills JL, Simpson JL, Driscoll SG, et al. Incidence of spontaneous abortion among normal women and insulin-dependent diabetic women whose pregnancies were identified within 21 days of conception. N Engl J Med 1988;319:1617–23.
[4] Mills JL, Fishl AR, Knopp RH, et al. Malformations in infants of diabetic mothers: problems in study design. Prev Med 1983;12:274–86.
[5] Jovanovic L, Peterson CM, Saxena BB, et al. Feasibility of maintaining normal glucose profiles in insulin-dependent pregnant diabetic women. Am J Med 1980;68:105–12.
[6] DeVeciana M, Major CA, Morgan MA, et al. Postprandial versus preprandial blood glucose monitoring in women with gestational diabetes mellitus requiring insulin therapy. N Engl J Med 1995;333:1237–41.
[7] Combs CA, Gunderson E, Kitzmiller JL, et al. Relationship of fetal macrosomia to maternal postprandial glucose control during pregnancy. Diabetes Care 1992;15:1251–7.
[8] Jovanovic L, Peterson CM, Reed GF, et al. Maternal postprandial glucose levels and infant birth weight: the diabetes in early pregnancy study. Am J Obstet Gynecol 1991;164:103–11.
[9] Jovanovic L. What is so bad about a big baby? [editorial] Diabetes Care 2001;24:1317–8.
[10] Challier JC, Haugel S, Desmaizieres V. Effects of insulin on glucose uptake and metabolism in the human placenta. J Clin Endocrinol Metab 1986;62:803–7.

[11] Boskovic R, Feig DS, Derewlany L, et al. Transfer of insulin lispro across the human placenta: in vitro perfusion studies. Diabetes Care 2003;26:1390–4.

[12] Menon RK, Cohen RM, Sperling MA, et al. Transplacental passage of insulin in pregnant women with insulin-dependent diabetes mellitus. Its role in fetal macrosomia. N Engl J Med 1990;323:309–15.

[13] Jovanovic L, Kitzmiller JL, Peterson CM. Randomized trial of human versus animal species insulin in diabetic pregnant women: improved glycemic control, not fewer antibodies to insulin, influences birth weight. Am J Obstet Gynecol 1992;167:1325–30.

[14] Moses RG, Lucas EM, Knights S. Gestational diabetes mellitus: at what time should the postprandial glucose level be monitored? Aust N Z J Obstet Gynecol 1999;39:457–60.

[15] Anderson JH Jr, Brunelle RL, Koivisto VA, et al. Reduction of postprandial hyperglycemia and frequency of hypoglycemia in IDDM patients on insulin-analogue treatment. Diabetes 1997;46:265–70.

[16] Fineberg SE, Rathbun MJ, Hufferd S, et al. Immunologic aspects of human proinsulin therapy. Diabetes 1988;37:276–80.

[17] Fineberg NS, Fineberg SE, Anderson JH, et al. Immunologic effects of insulin lispro Lys (B23), Pro (B29) human insulin in IDDM and NIDDM patients previously treated with insulin. Diabetes 1996;45:1750–4.

[18] Setter SM, Corbett CF, Campbell RK, et al. Insulin aspart: a new rapid-acting insulin analogue. Ann Pharmacother 2000;34:1423–31.

[19] Calle-Pascual AL, Bagazgoitia J, Calle JR, et al. Use of insulin lispro in pregnancy. Diabetes Nutr Metab 2003;13:173–7.

[20] Jovanovic L, Ilic S, Pettitt DJ, et al. The metabolic and immunologic effects of insulin lispro in gestational diabetes. Diabetes Care 1999;22:1422–6.

[21] Jovanovic L, Druzin M, Peterson CM. The effect of euglycemia on the outcome of pregnancy in insulin-dependent diabetics as compared to normal controls. Am J Med 1981;71:921–7.

[22] Jovanovic L, Mills Jl, Knopp RH, et al, the National Institute of Child Health and Human Development-Diabetes in Early Pregnancy Study Group. Declining insulin requirement in the late first trimester of diabetic pregnancy. Diabetes Care 2001;24:1130–6.

[23] Langer O, Yogev Y, Most O, et al. Gestational diabetes: the consequences of not treating. Am J Obstet Gynecol 2002;192:989–97.

[24] American Diabetes Association. Gestational diabetes mellitus (position statement). Diabetes Care 2004;27(Suppl 1):S88–90.

[25] Thompson DM, Dansereau J, Creed M, et al. Tight glucose control results in normal perinatal outcome in 150 patients with gestational diabetes. Obstet Gynecol 1994;83:362–6.

[26] Langer O, Mazze R. The relationship between large-for-gestational-age infants and glycemic control in women with gestational diabetes. Am J Obstet Gynecol 1988;159:1478–83.

[27] Metzger BE, Coustan DR. The Organizing Committee. Summary and recommendations of the Fourth International Workshop-Conference on Gestational Diabetes Mellitus. Diabetes Care 1998;21(Suppl 2):B161–7.

[28] Jovanovic L, editor. Medical management of pregnancy complicated by diabetes. Alexandria (VA): American Diabetes Association; 2000.

[29] Engelgau M, German R, Herman W, et al. The epidemiology of diabetes and pregnancy in the U.S. 1988. Diabetes Care 1995;18:1029–33.

[30] Persson B, Hanson U. Neonatal morbidities in gestational diabetes mellitus. Diabetes Care 1998;21(Suppl 2):B79–84.

[31] Hod M, Rabinerson D, Peled Y. Gestational diabetes mellitus: is it a clinical entity? Diabetes Rev 1995;3:603–13.

[32] Ogata ES. Perinatal morbidity in offspring of diabetic mothers. Diabetes Rev 1995;3:652–7.

[33] Langer O. Is normoglycemia the correct threshold to prevent complications in the pregnant diabetic patient? Diabetes Rev 1995;4:2–10.

[34] Platt MJ, Stanisstreet M, Casson IF, et al. St Vincent declaration 10 years on: outcomes of diabetic pregnancies. Diabet Med 2002;19:216–20.

[35] Bolli GB. Insulin treatment in type 1 diabetes. Endocr Pract 2006;12(Suppl 1):105–9.

[36] Ashwell SG, Gebbie J, Home PD. Optimal timing of injection of once-daily insulin glargine in people with type 1 diabetes using insulin lispro at meal-times. Diabet Med 2006;23:46–52.

[37] Guerci B, Sauvanet JP. Subcutaneous insulin: pharmacokinetic variability and glycemic variability. Diabetes Metab 2005;31(4 Pt 2):4S7–4S24.

[38] Wilinska ME, Chassin LJ, Schaller HC, et al. Insulin kinetics in type-I diabetes: continuous and bolus delivery of rapid acting insulin. IEEE Trans Biomed Eng 2005;52(1):3–12.

[39] Hirsch IB. Insulin analogues. N Engl J Med 2005;352(2):174–83.

[40] Heinemann L, Kapitza C, Starke AA, et al. Time-action profile of the insulin analogue B28Asp. Diabet Med 1996;13:683–4.

[41] Home PD, Lindholm A, Hylleberg B, et al. Improved glycemic control with insulin aspart: a multi-center randomized double-blind crossover trial in type 1 diabetic patients. UK Insulin Aspart Study Group. Diabetes Care 1998;21:1904–9.

[42] Home PD, Barriocanal L, Lindholm A. Comparative pharmacokinetics and pharmacodynamics of the novel rapid-acting insulin analogue, insulin aspart, in healthy volunteers. Eur J Clin Pharmacol 1999;55:199–203.

[43] Novo Nordisk Pharmaceutical Company. NovoLog Product Labeling Physicians' Desk Reference. 58th edition. Montvale (NJ): Thomson PDR; 2004. p. 2355–2359.

[44] Rave K, Klein O, Frick AD, et al. Advantage of premeal-injected insulin glulisine compared with regular human insulin in subjects with type 1 diabetes. Diabetes Care 2006;29(8): 1812–7.

[45] Hoogma RP, Schumicki D. Safety of insulin glulisine when given by continuous subcutaneous infusion using an external pump in patients with type 1 diabetes. Horm Metab Res 2006; 38(6):429–33.

[46] Anderson J, Bastyr E, Wishner K. Response to diamond and kormas. N Engl J Med 1997; 337:1009–12.

[47] Robinson DM, Wellington K. Insulin glulisine. Drugs 2006;66(6):861–9.

[48] Bhattacharyya A, Brown S, Huges S, et al. Insulin lispro and regular insulin in pregnancy. QJM 2001;94:255–60.

[49] Mecacci F, Carignani L, Cioni R, et al. Maternal metabolic control and perinatal outcome in women with gestational diabetes treated with regular or lispro insulin: comparison with non-diabetic pregnant women. Eur J Obstet Gynecol Reprod Biol 2003;11:19–24.

[50] Wyatt JW, Frias JL, Hoyme HE, et al. Congenital anomaly rate in offspring of pregestational diabetic women treated with insulin lispro during pregnancy. Diabet Med 2004; 21:2001–7.

[51] Garg SK, Frias JP, Anil S, et al. Insulin lispro therapy in pregnancies complicated by diabetes type 1: glycemic control and maternal and fetal outcomes. Endocr Pract 2003;9:187–93.

[52] Pettitt DJ, Ospina P, Kolaczynski J, et al. Comparison of an insulin analogue, insulin aspart, and regular human insulin with no insulin in gestational diabetes mellitus. Diabetes Care 2003;26:183–6.

[53] Hod M. for the Novorapid Insulin Trial of the Safety and Efficacy of Insulin Aspart for the Treatment of Type 1 Diabetic Women during Pregnancy. Study design. Presented at the European Association for the Study of Diabetes, 2005.

[54] Cypryk K, Sobczak M, Pertynska-Marczewska M, et al. Pregnancy complications and perinatal outcome in diabetic women treated with Humalog (insulin lispro) or regular human insulin during pregnancy. Med Sci Monit 2004;10(2):PI29–32.

[55] Carr KJ, Idama TO, Masson EA, et al. A randomised controlled trial of insulin lispro given before or after meals in pregnant women with type 1 diabetes—the effect on glycaemic excursion. J Obstet Gynaecol 2004;24(4):382–6.

[56] Masson EA, Patmore JE, Brash PD, et al. Pregnancy outcome in type 1 diabetes mellitus treated with insulin lispro (Humalog). Diabet Med 2003;20(1):46–50.

[57] Persson B, Swahn ML, Hjertberg R, et al. Insulin lispro therapy in pregnancies complicated by type 1 diabetes mellitus. Diabetes Res Clin Pract 2002;58(2):115–21.

[58] Loukovaara S, Immonen I, Teramo KA, et al. Progression of retinopathy during pregnancy in type 1 diabetic women treated with insulin lispro. Diabetes Care 2003;26(4):1193–8.

[59] Rosenstock J, Dailey G, Massi-Benedetti M, et al. Reduced hypoglycemia risk with insulin glargine: a meta-analysis comparing insulin glargine with human NPH insulin in type 2 diabetes. Diabetes Care 2005;28:950–5.

[60] Hofmann T, Horstmann G, Stammberger I. Evaluation of the reproductive toxicity and embryotoxicity of insulin glargine (LANTUS) in rats and rabbits. Int J Toxicol 2002;21:181–9.

[61] Devlin JT, Hothersall L, Wilkis JL. Use of insulin glargine during pregnancy in a type 1 diabetic woman. Diabetes Care 2002;25:1095–6.

[62] Porcellati F, Rossetti P, Pampanelli S, et al. Better long-term glycaemic control with the basal insulin glargine as compared with NPH in patients with type 1 diabetes mellitus given meal-time lispro insulin. Diabet Med 2004;21(11):1213–20.

[63] Di Cianni G, Volpe L, Lencioni C, et al. Use of insulin glargine during the first weeks of pregnancy in five type 1 diabetic women. Diabetes Care 2005;28:982–3.

[64] Holstein A, Plaschke A, Egberts EH. Use of insulin glargine during embryogenesis in a pregnant woman with type 1 diabetes. Diabet Med 2003;20:779–80.

[65] Caronna S, Cioni F, Dall'Aglio E, et al. Pregnancy and the long-acting insulin analogue: a case study. Acta Biomed Ateneo Parmense 2006;77(1):24–6.

[66] Torlone E, Gennarini A, Ricci NB, et al. Successful use of insulin glargine during entire pregnancy until delivery in six type 1 diabetic women. Eur J Obstet Gynecol Reprod Biol 2006 Jun 24; [Epub ahead of print].

[67] Dolci M, Mori M, Baccetti F. Use of glargine insulin before and during pregnancy in a woman with type 1 diabetes and Addison's disease. Diabetes Care 2005;28(8):2084–5.

[68] Wooldrenrink JM, van Loon AJ, Storms F, et al. Use of insulin glargine during pregnancy in seven type 1 diabetic women. Diabetes Care 2005;28:2394–5.

[69] Graves DE, White JC, Kirk JK. The use of insulin glargine with gestational diabetes mellitus. Diabetes Care 2006;29(2):471–2.

[70] Hamilton-Wessler M, Ader M, Dea M, et al. Mechanism of protracted metabolic effects of fatty acid acylated insulin, NN304, in dogs: retention of NN304 by albumin. Diabetologia 1999;42:1254–63.

[71] Kurtzhals P, Havelund S, Jonassen I, et al. Albumin binding of insulins acylated with fatty acids: characterization of the ligand-protein interaction and correlation between binding affinity and timing of the insulin effect in vivo. Biochem J 1995;312(Pt 3):725–31.

[72] Whittingham JL, Havelund S, Jonassen I. Crystal structure of a prolonged-acting insulin with albumin-binding properties. Biochemistry 1997;36:2826–31.

[73] Home PD, Bartley P, Russell-Jones D, et al. Insulin detemir offers improved glycemic control compared with NPH insulin in people with Type 1 diabetes: a randomized clinical trial. Diabetes Care 2004;27:1081–7.

[74] Hermansen K, Fontaine P, Kukolja KK, et al. Insulin analogues (insulin detemir and insulin aspart) versus traditional human insulins (NPH insulin and regular human insulin) in basal-bolus therapy for patients with Type 1 diabetes. Diabetologia 2004;47:622–9.

[75] Druckmann R, Rohr UD. IGF-1 in gynaecology and obstetrics: update 2002. Maturitas 2002;41(Suppl 1):S65–83.

[76] Mandl M, J.Haas J, Bischof P, et al. Serum-dependent effects of IGF-I and insulin on proliferation and invasion of human first trimester trophoblast cell models. Histochem Cell Biol 2002;117:391–9.

[77] The Diabetes Control and Complications Trial Research Group. Effect of pregnancy on microvascular complications in the diabetes control and complications trial. Diabetes Care 2000;23:1084–91.

[78] Lacroix MC, Guibourdenche J, Frendo JL, et al. Human placental growth hormone–a review. Placenta 2002;23(Suppl A):S87–94.

[79] De Meyts P, Whittaker J. Structural biology of insulin and IGF1 receptors: implications for drug design. Nat Rev Drug Discov 2002;1:769–83.

[80] Drejer K. The bioactivity of insulin analogues from in vitro receptor binding to in vivo glucose uptake. Diabetes Metab Rev 1992;8:259–85.

[81] Bahr M, Kolter T, Seipke G, et al. Growth promoting and metabolic activity of the human insulin analogue [GlyA21,ArgB31,ArgB32] insulin (HOE 901) in muscle cells. Eur J Pharmacol 1997;320:259–65.

[82] Kurtzhals P, Schaffer L, Sorensen A, et al. Correlations of receptor binding and metabolic and mitogenic potencies of insulin analogues designed for clinical use. Diabetes 2000;49: 999–1005.

[83] Ciaraldi TP, Carter L, Seipke G, et al. Effects of the long-acting insulin analogue insulin glargine on cultured human skeletal muscle cells: comparisons to insulin and IGF-I. J Clin Endocrinol Metab 2001;86:5838–47.

[84] Sheth BP. Does pregnancy accelerate the rate of progression of diabetic retinopathy? Curr Diab Rep 2002;2:327–30.

[85] Henricsson M, Berntorp K, Berntorp E, et al. Progression of retinopathy after improved metabolic control in type 2 diabetic patients. Relation to IGF-1 and hemostatic variables. Diabetes Care 1999;22:1944–9.

[86] Phelps RL, Sakol P, Metzger BE, et al. Changes in diabetic retinopathy during pregnancy. Correlations with regulation of hyperglycemia. Arch Ophthalmol 1986;104:1806–10.

[87] Chew EY, Mills JL, Metzger BE, et al. Metabolic control and progression of retinopathy. The Diabetes in Early Pregnancy Study. National Institute of Child Health and Human Development Diabetes in Early Pregnancy Study. Diabetes Care 1995;18:631–7.

[88] DCCT Study Group and KROC Study Group. Diabetic retinopathy after two years of intensified insulin treatment. Follow-up of the Kroc Collaborative Study. The Kroc Collaborative Study Group. JAMA 1988;260:37–41.

[89] DCCT Study Group and KROC Study Group. The effect of intensive treatment of diabetes on the development and progression of long-term complications in insulin-dependent diabetes mellitus. The Diabetes Control and Complications Trial Research Group. N Engl J Med 1993;329:977–86.

[90] Early worsening of diabetic retinopathy in the Diabetes Control and Complications Trial. Arch Ophthalmol 1998;116:874–86.

[91] Kondo T, Vicent D, Suzuma K, et al. Knockout of insulin and IGF-1 receptors on vascular endothelial cells protects against retinal neovascularization. J Clin Invest 2003;111:1835–42.

[92] Kitzmiller JL, Main E, Ward B, et al. Insulin lispro and the development of proliferative diabetic retinopathy during pregnancy. Diabetes Care 1999;22:874–6.

[93] Buchbinder A, Miodovnik M, McElvy S, et al. Is insulin lispro associated with the development or progression of diabetic retinopathy during pregnancy? Am J Obstet Gynecol 2000; 183:1162–5.

[94] Jovanovic L. Retinopathy risk: what is responsible? Hormones, hyperglycemia, or Humalog? Response to Kitzmiller, et al. Diabetes Care 1999;22:846–8.

ELSEVIER
SAUNDERS

Obstet Gynecol Clin N Am
34 (2007) 293–307

OBSTETRICS AND
GYNECOLOGY
CLINICS
OF NORTH AMERICA

# Diabetic-Associated Stillbirth: Incidence, Pathophysiology, and Prevention

## Donald J. Dudley, MD

*Department of Obstetrics and Gynecology, University of Texas Health Science Center
at San Antonio, 7703 Floyd Curl Drive, San Antonio, TX 78229, USA*

An increased risk for stillbirth has been a recognized potential complication of diabetes for over 100 years. This increased risk is most commonly associated with insulin-requiring pregestational diabetes, but may also be evident in other forms of diabetes complicating pregnancy. This article focuses on the association of stillbirth with diabetes, the potential pathophysiology of stillbirth in pregnancies complicated by diabetes, and strategies to reduce the risk of stillbirth in women who have diabetes.

### Definitions

For the purposes of this review, pregestational diabetes may include type 1 or type 2 diabetes. Gestational diabetes is that recognized only during pregnancy after specific testing. Although some cases of type 2 diabetes may be detected during pregnancy, the specific diagnosis may not be clear. These instances will be considered as gestational diabetes because of the lack of clarity of diagnosis before the pregnancy.

Stillbirth is generally defined as fetal death after 20 weeks of gestation. One problem that has plagued epidemiologic and pathophysiologic studies of stillbirth has been the lack of precise definition of stillbirth [1]. Some authorities and state health departments only include birth weights less than 350 g, or less than 500 g, or heel–toe lengths of xx cm. This lack of precision in the definition of stillbirth continues to cause confusion in the interpretation of studies regarding stillbirth. Other terms for stillbirth include *fetal death, intrauterine fetal death, fetal demise,* and *intrauterine fetal*

---

Supported in part by a grant from the National Institutes of Health: HD.
*E-mail address:* dudleyd@uthscsa.edu

doi:10.1016/j.ogc.2007.03.001
*obgyn.theclinics.com*

*demise*. For purposes of clarity, in this review, the terms *stillbirth* and *fetal death* are used interchangeably.

The term *perinatal mortality rate* is defined as the number of stillbirths after 20 weeks gestation plus the number of infant deaths up to 28 days of life. One limiting aspect of past studies on the contribution of diabetes to the incidence of stillbirth is a lack of precision in terminology. Many studies report perinatal mortality and do not specifically address stillbirth. Understanding the attributable risk for diabetes and stillbirth is thus limited by lack of precision.

### Historical perspective

Prior to the discovery of insulin, successful pregnancy was rare in women who had pregestational diabetes. In women who achieved pregnancy, the perinatal mortality rate approximated 65% [2]. Notably, however, maternal mortality was exceedingly high, approaching 30%; thus, concerns regarding the perinatal mortality rate were superceded by maternal concerns. With the discovery and then the clinical use of insulin, maternal mortality rates declined dramatically, and attention could be turned to improving the perinatal mortality rate.

Even with improved maternal outcomes, fetal death rates proved to be more intransigent until the 1960s (Fig. 1). With improved prenatal care, including fetal surveillance techniques, aggressive blood sugar control, sonography, timely labor induction, and advanced neonatal care, the rate of fetal death in women who have diabetes has decreased dramatically [3].

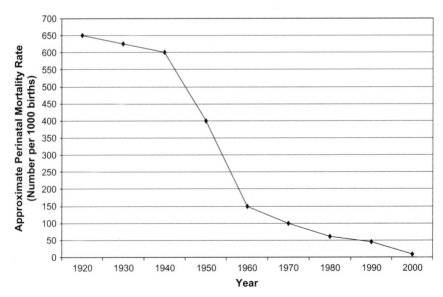

Fig. 1. Estimated rate of stillbirth in diabetic women: 1920–2000. These estimates of the stillbirth rate in diabetic women are based on a summary of the reported literature.

## Epidemiology of stillbirth

Fetal deaths have declined over the past 50 years. In the 1950s, fetal death rates were reported as high as 20/1000 births. However, according to the most recent National Center for Health Statistic report from 2003 [1], fetal deaths occurred in 6.23/1000 births. However, this figure has been declined slowly over the past 20 years, while the number of infant deaths has declined by over 30% in that same time period [4]. Most of the decline in fetal deaths has occurred in gestational ages of greater than 28 weeks, perhaps reflecting improved fetal surveillance.

In the 2003 NCHS report [1], a higher risk of fetal death occurs in non-Hispanic black women (11.56/1000 births), teenagers, women over the age of 35, unmarried women (8.25/1000 births), and in multiple gestations (twins, 16.52/1000 births). Clearly, a better understanding of the causes of stillbirth is needed to decrease the fetal death rates in this country. To accomplish this, the National Institutes of Health created the Stillbirth Collaborative Research Network to study to the epidemiology and causes of fetal death in five defined geographic catchment areas. This landmark hypothesis–driven study will provide critically needed information to address the problem of fetal death, and hypotheses to study the potential role of diabetes as a cause of fetal death have been proposed.

Other risk factors for stillbirth that may be important in the consideration of stillbirth in diabetic women included obesity, prior cesarean delivery, congenital birth defects, and fetal growth restriction [5]. Maternal obesity is associated with a doubled risk for stillbirth (odds ratio of 2.8) [6]. Women who have diabetes are much more likely to undergo cesarean delivery, and this operative delivery is associated with a modestly increased risk for stillbirth (hazard ratio of 2.27). Congenital fetal abnormalities are associated with an increased risk for stillbirth, and diabetic women are two to three times more likely to have an infant who has birth defects. A particularly strong risk factor for stillbirth is fetal growth restriction for any number of maternal or fetal conditions and in particular diabetes associated with vascular complications. Recently, Gardosi and colleagues [7] have postulated that fetuses not meeting their growth potential are a strong risk factor for fetal death.

*Stillbirth in women who have type 1 diabetes mellitus*

Pregestational diabetes is commonly divided into type 1 and type 2 diabetes. Both types are associated with an increased risk for stillbirth in pregnant women. Type 1 diabetes is associated with a three to five times increased risk for stillbirth (Table 1). In Denmark from 1990 to 2000, Lauenborg and colleagues [8] reported that women who have type 1 diabetes had an incidence of stillbirth of 18/1000 pregnancies. Notably, an explainable cause was found in approximately one third of cases having nothing to do with diabetes. Of those women who have unexplained stillbirth,

Table 1
Epidemiology of stillbirth in type 1 diabetics

| Country | Years of study | Sample size | Rate/1000 births | Relative risk | Reference |
|---------|----------------|-------------|------------------|---------------|-----------|
| Denmark | 1990–2000 | 1361 | 18 | — | [8] |
| Denmark | 1993–1999 | 1218 | 21 | 6.2 | [9] |
| Scotland | 1979–1995 | 1112 | 25 | 4.7 | [10] |
| Scotland | 1998–1999 | 273 | 18.5 | 3.6 | [11] |
| UK | 1990–1994 | 462 | 25 | 5.0 | [12] |
| UK | 2002–2003 | 1707 | 25.8 | 4.5 | [13] |
| USA | 1995–1997 | 271,691 | 5.9 | 1.5 | [14] |

75% (9/12) were associated with hyperglycemia and elevated hemoglobin A1C levels (>7.5%). Also, other Danish investigators reported from eight centers managing 1218 pregnancies from 1993 to 1999 [9]. Their stillbirth rate was 28/1000 births compared with a rate in the general population of 4.5/1000 (relative risk 6.2). As with other studies, serious adverse outcomes were associated with poor metabolic control.

Similarly, a recent report from Scotland [10] found the incidence of stillbirth to be 25/1000 births of women who have pregestational insulin-requiring diabetes from 1979 to 1995. The overall stillbirth rate was 4.7 times higher than that found in the general population. Of note, the risk for stillbirth decreased with increasing gestational age. In a later study from Scotland [11], the Scottish Diabetes in Pregnancy Group reported on a cohort of 273 pregnancies ascertained over 1 year (1998–1999). They found a stillbirth rate of 18.5/1000 births, with a relative risk of 3.6 over the stillbirth rate in all Scottish births over the same time period.

In the United Kingdom, Casson and colleagues [12] reported on 462 pregnancies in 355 women who have type 1 diabetes from 1990 to 1994. The stillbirth rate was 25/1000 births, compared with a stillbirth rate in the general population of 5/1000 (relative risk 5). Also in the United Kingdom, a sample of 1707 type 1 diabetic women was ascertained from 2002 to 2003 with a stillbirth rate of 25.8/1000 births being reported [13]. The stillbirth rate in the general population was 5.7/1000 births, yielding a rate ratio of 4.5, a figure consistent with other reports.

Outcomes in the United States seem to be much better than these other reports. Mondestin and colleagues [14] recently reported National Center for Health Statistics data that put the fetal death for women who have diabetes at 5.9/1000, and an overall fetal death rate in the nondiabetic population of 4.0/1000 births. One weakness in this study is that gestational, pregestational, type 1, and type 2 diabetes are not discriminated in the reporting. Therefore, we cannot directly assess the risk posed in the overall United States population from each type of diabetes. Regardless, the risk for fetal death in type 1 diabetes seems to be higher than the general population, and history has shown us that uncontrolled type 1 diabetes is a strong risk factor for fetal death.

## Stillbirth in women who have type 2 diabetes mellitus

Similar to type 1 diabetes, women who have type 2 diabetes have an increased risk for stillbirth (Table 2). However, the extent of this increased risk is variable with different populations.

In a study from New Zealand, Cundy and colleagues [15] reported on 434 pregnancies complicated by type 2 diabetes. They found that the risk of fetal death was much greater in type 2 diabetes than type 1 diabetes (approximately 34/1000 births versus approximately 12/1000 births). Women who have type 2 diabetes had much worse glucose control, and this was a significant risk factor for fetal death. The authors suggested that this may be due to the increased risk posed by obesity, essential hypertension, and maternal age. Women who had newly diagnosed type 2 diabetics had significantly worse outcomes. Similarly, Clausen and colleagues [16] found that women who had type 2 diabetes had worse outcomes than women who had type 1 diabetes, with perinatal mortality rates of 67/1000 and 17/1000, respectively.

In the United Kingdom, Dunne and colleagues [17] noted that in 182 women who had type 2 diabetes, only two stillbirths occurred (12.2/1000 births). This figure compared with national data on stillbirths in the general population (5.4/1000) yielding a relative risk of 2.3. In the study previously noted from Macintosh and colleagues [13] of 652 women who had type 2 diabetes, the stillbirth rate was similar to that noted in women who had type 1 diabetes, 29.2/1000 births. Compared to normal pregnancy, the relative risk for stillbirth in women who had type 2 diabetes was 5.1.

## Stillbirth in women who have gestational diabetes mellitus

Women who develop gestational diabetes mellitus (GDM) seem to have an increased risk for stillbirth, although the data to support this observation are not as strong as the increased risk noted for type 1 and type 2 diabetes.

In 1973, O'Sullivan and colleagues [18] reported a higher perinatal mortality rate in women who had GDM. In this study of 187 women who had GDM, a perinatal mortality rate of 64/1000 births was noted (12/187). This increased risk seemed to predominate in women over the age of 25. No data regarding the nature of the increased mortality rates were presented. White and Beischer [19] reported a perinatal mortality rate of 16/1000 births in women who have GDM. A stillbirth rate of 7/1000 births could be gleaned from this report, and the main causes of perinatal mortality included

Table 2
Epidemiology of stillbirth in type 2 diabetics

| Country | Years of study | Sample size | Rate/1000 births | Relative risk | Reference |
|---------|---------------|-------------|------------------|---------------|-----------|
| UK | 1990–2002 | 182 | 12.2 | 2.3 | [17] |
| UK | 2002–2003 | 652 | 29.2 | 5.1 | [13] |
| New Zealand | 1985–1997 | 434 | 34[a] | 2.8[a] | [15] |

[a] Estimated rate.

congenital anomalies, respiratory distress with prematurity, and intrauterine hypoxia. In a follow-up study, Beischer and colleagues [20] found that routine screening for GDM could significantly improve perinatal outcome. In a large population of 116,303 pregnancies screened for diabetes, diagnosed GDM was found to have an increased risk for perinatal mortality (adjusted odds ratio of 1.53). Women who were diagnosed retrospectively had a higher odds ratio of 2.31, and women who were not screened continued to have a higher odds ratio for stillbirth (2.21).

More recently, Aberg and colleagues [21], from Sweden, reported that women who were subsequently diagnosed with GDM had a higher incidence of stillbirth in preceding pregnancies, suggesting that these women had undiagnosed GDM in these pregnancies ending in fetal death. In this case–control study, the odds ratio for fetal death in the preceding pregnancy was 1.56, with a stillbirth rate of 15/1000 compared with the normal control stillbirth rate of 6.5/1000. Similarly, Wood and colleagues [22] found that women who were considered "prediabetic" (ie, a pregnancy before the diagnosis of diabetes) had a higher risk for stillbirth than a nondiabetic control population (19.7/1000 births versus 5.5/1000 births). Women who had pregestational diabetes had a stillbirth rate of 33.7/1000. The authors suggest that these women who were considered prediabetic were actually misclassified and had overt diabetes during their studied pregnancy.

Girz and colleagues [23] reported that despite an intensive monitoring system for women who had GDM, the stillbirth rate was 7.7/1000 compared with a nondiabetic control population of 4.8/1000. This increased rate of stillbirth was noted despite an intensive fetal surveillance program and aggressive obstetric management of abnormal fetal testing.

A recent study by Challis and colleagues [24] in Mozambique found no association of gestational diabetes or impaired glucose tolerance in a population where fetal death is common (approximately 5% of all pregnancies). In this study, the authors found that GDM complicated 11% of 109 women with fetal death, and 7% of matched women without GDM, a nonsignificant difference.

Although one finds it difficult to find a consistently increased risk for stillbirth in women who have gestational diabetes, there does appear to be increased risk; although this risk appears to be smaller than that found in women who have type 1 and type 2 diabetes. Many studies are difficult to interpret because fetal and neonatal deaths are not analyzed separately. Also, small sample sizes limit many studies. For example, the study by Langer and colleagues [25], perhaps one of the largest reports regarding GDM during pregnancy, found that women who had untreated GDM had a stillbirth rate of 5.4/1000, whereas nondiabetic control patients had a stillbirth rate of 1.8/1000. However, because of the small numbers and large confidence intervals, these differences were not statistically significant. Regardless, diagnosis of GDM and aggressive management seems to improve perinatal outcomes and lessen, although not eliminate, the increased risk for stillbirth.

## Causes of stillbirth

When considering stillbirth in women who have diabetes, one must remember that there are multiple causes of stillbirth for all women, and that hyperglycemia is but one cause. In a recent review from the Stillbirth Collaborative Research Network, Silver and colleagues [26] note that the causes of stillbirth are varied and in many cases unexplained. In current practice, a cause may be ascertained in only 50% of cases of stillbirth, whereas a more detailed evaluation may uncover a cause in up to 90% of cases. The causes of stillbirth may be classified according to a wide variety of classification schemes, all of which reflect a specific bias depending on the perspective of the investigator (eg, pathologic, obstetric, vascular, and so forth). As such, none are completely satisfactory, but these different classifications do provide for at least some common language for investigation and discussion.

Stillbirth may be caused by maternal or fetal conditions, and may be the result of maternal–fetal interactions. Commonly recognized causes of stillbirth include fetal malformations, fetal aneuploidy, placental malformations, placental insufficiency, fetal infection, feto-maternal hemorrhage, maternal hypertension, systemic maternal infection and sepsis, and maternal vascular disease (eg, systemic lupus erythematosus, antiphospholipid syndrome).

## Pathophysiology of stillbirth in women who have diabetes

General consensus holds that hyperglycemia and poor glucose control contributes significantly to the events that lead to fetal death in women who have diabetes [27]. However, other causes of stillbirth cannot be discounted, and studies of fetal death in diabetic women that include a detailed analysis of the causes of fetal death find that uncontrolled hyperglycemia probably accounts for approximately half of all fetal deaths. Congenital anomalies, infection, and other known causes of stillbirth account for the other half. As with nondiabetic women who suffer stillbirth, a significant proportion remains unexplained. Even though hyperglycemia is a potential cause for stillbirth, other causes account for a significant proportion of stillbirths. Therefore, women who have diabetes who suffer fetal death should be offered a complete evaluation to determine the cause of the fetal death, including autopsy, placental evaluation, and laboratory evaluation [26].

### Human studies

The cause of fetal death in women who have pregestational diabetes is not clear. Historically, the likely pathophysiology for the deaths has been attributed to undetected hyperglycemia and ketoacidosis [27]. Past reports have noted perinatal mortality death rates of 50% to 90% in women in ketoacidosis. However, few data from women are available to provide insight into how diabetes, and in particular hyperglycemia, contribute to the pathophysiologic events leading to fetal death. Unnoticed hypoglycemia has been suggested as a possible cause, but there are not compelling data available to support this concept.

Infusion of glucose into normal and diabetic pregnant women during labor has been associated with neonatal hypoxia and acidosis [28]. In a study of 28 type 1 diabetic women whereby fetal blood sampling was completed between 20 and 40 weeks gestation, Bradley and colleagues [29] noted that there were deviations in fetal blood pH and plasma lactate with significant acidosis in the third trimester. The authors note that some fetuses in the third trimester are significantly acidotic, and that this may contribute to so-called "unexplained fetal death" in diabetic women in the third trimester.

These findings indicate that at least some cases of fetal death in women who have pregestational diabetes fetal hyperglycemia may be associated with accumulations of fetal lactic acid as a result of hyperinsulinemia leading to anaerobic metabolism with consequent hypoxia and acidosis.

*Animal studies*

Several different animal models have been used to explore the fetal risk of diabetes, including rats, sheep, and Rhesus monkeys. In particular, rats seem to be an excellent model for the study of diabetes during pregnancy. In sheep, hyperglycemia, when paired with hypoxia, resulted in a greater risk for fetal death [30]. In Rhesus monkeys, hypoxia combined with hyperglyemia was particularly lethal [31], leading to excessive accumulations of lactic acid in the central nervous system of these animals.

More recent animal studies indicate that diabetic pregnancy is associated with significantly greater oxidative stress. Damasceno and colleagues [32] studied antioxidant activity in the streptozotocin-induced diabetic pregnant rat model. They found that oxidative stress occurs in these animals, potentially resulting in alterations of maternal homeostasis that may explain the increased risk for fetal malformations and pregnancy loss.

Recent studies from Uppsala University, led by Ericksson, provide some insights into the oxidative stresses provoked by drug-induced diabetes in pregnant rats. In early studies by Wentzel and colleagues [33], they found that increased substrate availability (hyperglycemia) led to enhanced oxidative stress, and increased supply of nutrients to the uterus and developing embryos resulted in fewer implantations and higher malformation rates. Using this model in a subsequent study, these investigators supplemented the diet of diabetic rats with two antioxidants, vitamin C and E, and found that animals supplemented with high concentrations of these antioxidants had malformation rates similar to nondiabetic rats [34]. These data indicated that antioxidant treatment diminished damage associated with oxygen radicals, and might be a potential therapy to reduce birth defects and fetal loss in human diabetic pregnancies. In a separate recent study, Gareskog and colleagues [35] reported that these diabetic rats showed evidence of increased apoptosis, or programmed cell death, in embryos exposed to the diabetic environment. They speculated that these apoptotic events may contribute to dysmorphogeneis and fetal loss in these pregnancies.

Studies such as these are critical to understanding the pathophysiology of fetal loss during diabetic pregnancy. They inform future studies in humans to determine if oxidative stress contributes to fetal death and the possibility that antioxidants may contribute to improved perinatal outcome. Caution must be exercised; recent studies on the role of antioxidants in the prevention of pre-eclampsia showed no efficacy and an increased risk for fetal loss [36].

## Prevention of stillbirth in diabetic pregnancies

Key to the prevention of fetal death in women who have pregestational diabetes is comprehensive multidisciplinary care with aggressive blood sugar control. The care team, led by an experienced perinatologist, should include internists, ophthalmologists, high-risk obstetric nurses, nutritionists, social workers, and a contemporary laboratory for specialized testing when indicated [27]. A new concept for complex patient care, patient navigation, holds promise for more effective and efficient care with improved perinatal outcomes [37].

### Comprehensive care

Temple and colleagues [38] showed conclusively that preconceptional care with intensive multidisciplinary management of type 1 diabetes is associated with improved pregnancy outcomes. In their cohort of 290 pregnancies, women who sought preconceptional care had markedly decreased risk of adverse pregnancy outcomes and very preterm deliveries (2.9 versus 10.2% in the no preconceptional care cohort for adverse pregnancy outcomes, 5.0 versus 14.2% for preterm births). Clearly, improved blood sugar with decreased hemoglobin A1C levels resulted in improved pregnancy outcomes for this cohort.

Johnstone and colleagues [39] reported that perinatal mortality in women who have type 1 diabetes declined significantly over the past 40 years, from 225/1000 births in the decade of 1960 to 1969 to 10/1000 births in the 1990s. They attributed this remarkable improvement to advances in obstetric and neonatal management and to improved blood glucose control. However, birth weight did not change over the 40 years, indicating that better understanding of the role of diabetes in determining birth weight is necessary before the problem of macrosomia can be addressed through prenatal care interventions.

*Achieve and maintain euglycemia*

One key method to prevent stillbirth in diabetic women is to scrupulously control blood sugar readings and achieve euglycemia. Many high-risk centers use a multidisciplinary approach including perinatologists, dieticians, and high-risk prenatal nursing staff to aggressively monitor glycemic control. In some cases, so-called "aggressive management" of diabetes has resulted in salutary outcomes for these women [40]. At the University of Texas Health Science Center at San Antonio, diabetic women are encouraged to check blood sugar readings seven times per day, and a remarkable percentage of women achieve this level of monitoring. Increased monitoring is associated with fewer stillbirths, less risk for macrosomia, and less risk for injury to the neonate at the time of delivery.

One hallmark of aggressive blood sugar control is the timely and intensive use of insulin, particularly in pregestational diabetic women. Multiple doses of insulin (more than twice a day) has been shown to provide for better control of blood sugars with hyperglycemic and hypoglycemic episodes. Reducing extremes in blood sugar readings may be an important tool to reduce the risk of stillbirth. Unfortunately, first-trimester hemoglobin A1C levels have low specificity and sensitivity in predicting adverse pregnancy outcomes [41], although high hemoglobin A1C levels are in general associated with poorer outcomes [42]. No specific discriminatory value for hemoglobin A1C has been described, and there are no clear cut-offs below which further improvement in blood sugar control has no effect on pregnancy outcome.

In general, oral hypoglycemic agents should be reserved for women who have gestational diabetes who do not meet with success in obtaining euglycemia with diet alone [43]. Currently, data are insufficient to conclude that the use of oral hypoglycemic agents reduces the risk of stillbirth in women who have GDM.

*Antepartum fetal surveillance*

One aspect of prenatal care that may contribute to reducing the risk for stillbirth is antenatal fetal monitoring. Current recommendations are that all women should be counseled regarding the use of fetal movement (fetal kick counts). While there is a paucity of data to show that these measures conclusively reduce the risk of stillbirth in diabetic women, this simple noninvasive technique seems reasonable, is inexpensive, and may have other benefits such as improved maternal bonding.

A mainstay of antenatal fetal surveillance is nonstress testing (NST), with or without determinations of amniotic fluid volume, and biophysical profile. Kjos and colleagues [44] described obstetric outcomes in 2134 women who have all types of diabetes using an antepartum fetal surveillance program of twice weekly NSTs with amniotic fluid volume determinations. They found that no stillbirths occurred within 4 days of the last antepartum testing, and that 85 women required cesarean delivery for fetal distress. Predictive factors for emergent cesarean delivery for nonreassuring fetal tracings included spontaneous decelerations, nonreactive NSTs, and both findings together. Using this testing scheme, these investigators were able to accomplish a salutary stillbirth rate of 1.4/1000. Given these results, most centers currently use weekly or twice weekly NSTs to monitor fetal well-being in women who have all forms of diabetes.

In a more recent study, Brecher and colleagues [45] reported a retrospective case–control study in which 1935 women who had all types of diabetes experienced weekly or twice weekly NSTs or biophysical profiles. They found that women who experienced stillbirths were more likely to have suboptimal glucose control and a greater time interval from their last fetal surveillance testing, as well as delivery at less than 37 weeks and birth weights less than 2500 g. Overall, they found a corrected perimortality rate of 4.1/1000 births.

Landon and Vickers [46], however, challenge the need for routine antepartum surveillance in women who have well-controlled diabetes and the absence of vascular complications. In such women, the need for intervention for abnormal testing is rare and is often presaged by difficulties in obtaining euglycemia. Further, these authors note the lack of data supporting antepartum testing in women who have GDM. Currently, most centers perform some form of antenatal testing for women who have GDM; there is a paucity of data and well-controlled trials showing efficacy of testing in these women.

A more recent addition to the armamentarium of studies to monitor fetal condition is Doppler velocimetry of the fetal or maternal vessels. Gradations of abnormal fetal blood velocity are associated with an increased risk for fetal acidemia. As placental resistance increases, fetal umbilical blood flow becomes increasingly retrograde, such that reversed end diastolic blood flow is a strong predictor of subsequent fetal death. Yoon and colleagues [47] reported that abnormalities of Doppler velocimetry were strongly associated with fetal acidosis and hypercarbia, but not hypoxemia. Further, they found that umbilical artery Doppler velocimetry was more sensitive than biophysical profile for fetal academia and hypercarbia. Reece and colleagues [48] found that in pregnant diabetic women, elevations of the systolic/diastolic ratio noted on Doppler velocimetry of the fetal umbilical artery was significantly associated with maternal vasculopathy associated with hypertension and renal insufficiency, as well as intrauterine growth restriction and neonatal metabolic complications, but not hyperglycemia.

In a comparison of NST, biophysical profile, and umbilical artery Doppler velocimetry, Bracero and colleagues [49] reported that Doppler studies better identified a subgroup of diabetic pregnancies that ended adversely than NSTs or biophysical profiles. The relative risk for adverse pregnancy outcome with abnormal Doppler studies, as reported by systolic/diastolic ratio, was 2.6, as opposed to a relative risk for abnormal NSTs or biophysical profiles of 1.7 each. The incidence of stillbirth was too rare in this study to compare the rates of stillbirth, thus surrogate markers for increased risk of stillbirth (eg, fetal growth restriction, fetal metabolic abnormalities) were used as a surrogate for fetal death. In a follow-up study [50], these same investigators found that umbilical Doppler velocimetry paired with hemoglobin A1C was much more predictive of adverse pregnancy outcome. Of those women who had abnormal Doppler studies and glycemic control, 96% had an adverse pregnancy outcome.

Although Doppler studies may identify women who are destined to have adverse pregnancy outcome, the sensitivity and specificity of abnormal testing is low. In 104 diabetic pregnancies, Wong and colleagues [51] found that Doppler studies had a sensitivity of 35%, specificity of 94%, positive predictive value of 80%, and negative predictive value of 68%. Only 30% of women in this study who had an adverse pregnancy outcome had abnormal Doppler studies. These authors concluded that Doppler studies were poor at predicting adverse pregnancy outcomes.

Pregnant women who have diabetes appear to have improved outcomes with some form of antepartum surveillance. However, the best methods, the best timing interval for testing, the optimal gestational age to begin testing, and the more accurate interpretations of the testing are still in evolution. Perhaps the most important lesson to learn is that antepartum fetal testing, no matter the form, seems to improve perinatal outcome to a modest to significant degree.

## Timing of delivery

The timing of delivery of the diabetic pregnant woman is key to improved outcomes. Obviously, the goal is to deliver a living infant, with an acceptable risk of cesarean delivery. Given the critical nature of this decision, many centers have developed algorithms to aid in the decision making regarding delivery. Common indications for delivery include an apparent inability to adhere to treatment regimens, hyperglycemia despite intensive efforts to gain control, abnormal fetal testing (NST, biophysical profiles, Doppler velocimetry), fetal growth restriction (less than 10% in women who have diabetes), and suspected fetal macrosomia. The prenatal diagnosis of fetal macrosomia is particularly problematic, and current recommendations are that fetuses of diabetic women who have estimated fetal weights of greater than 4500 g should be delivered by cesarean section [52]. The current practice at University of Texas Health Science Center at San Antonio to deliver with an estimated fetal weight of greater than 4250 g is based on retrospective studies of the specific population delivering through their program [53].

Regardless, one of the goals of the antenatal care program is to provide data regarding the diabetic pregnancy to inform the perinatologist or obstetrician as to the optimal timing of delivery to ensure the best possible neonatal outcome, with the prevention of stillbirth of critical importance in this decision.

Once the decision to induce labor rather than proceed with cesarean has been made, intrapartum monitoring is routinely employed in the hopes of ensuring the best possible pregnancy outcome with the lowest risk for cerebral palsy. Unfortunately, intrapartum fetal monitoring has not realized this goal [54]. However, most authorities agree that intrapartum fetal monitoring can decrease the risk for intrapartum stillbirth. In particular, intrapartum fetal monitoring should be employed in women who have diabetes, along with scrupulous control of maternal blood sugars during the course of labor.

## Summary

Diabetes, and in particularly pregestational diabetes with attendant vascular complications, is clearly a significant risk factor for stillbirth. However, a comprehensive prenatal care program, including perinatologists, dieticians, prenatal nurses, labor and delivery nurses and personnel, and social workers, can significantly improve pregnancy outcomes and decrease the risk for stillbirth in this vulnerable population that is approaching stillbirth rates that characterize normal pregnancies. An organized multidisciplinary approach to management of the diabetic pregnancy is essential for the success of the pregnancy.

## References

[1] MacDorman MF, Hoyert DL, Martin JA, et al. Fetal and perinatal mortality, United States, 2003. National vital statistics reports; vol. 55, no. (6). Hyattsville (MD): National Center for Health Statistics, 2007.

[2] Williams J. The clinical significance of glycosuria in pregnancy women. Am J Med Sci 1909; 137:1.

[3] Jovanovic L, Peterson CM. Management of the pregnant, insulin-dependent diabetic woman. Diabetes Care 1980;3:63–8.

[4] Silver RM. Fetal death. Obstet Gynecol 2007;109:153–67.

[5] Smith GCS. Predicting antepartum stillbirth. Curr Opin Obstet Gynecol 2006;18:625–30.

[6] Kristensen J, Vetergaard M, Wisborg K, et al. Pre-pregnancy weight and the risk of stillbirth and neonatal death. Br J Obstet Gynecol 2005;112:403–8.

[7] Gardosi J, Mul T, Mongelli M, et al. Analysis of birthweight and gestational age in antepartum stillbirths. Br J Obstet Gynaecol 1998;105:524–30.

[8] Lauenborg J, Mathiesen E, Ovesen P, et al. Audit on stillbirths in women with pregestational type 1 diabetes. Diabetes Care 2003;26:1385–9.

[9] Jensen D, Damm P, Moelsted-Pedersen L, et al. Outcomes in type 1 diabetic pregnancies. Diabetes Care 2004;27:2819–23.

[10] dos Santos Silva I, Higgins C, Swerdlow AJ, et al. Birthweight and other pregnancy outcomes in a cohort of women with pregestational insulin-treated diabetes mellitus, Scotland, 1979–1995. Diabet Med 2005;22:440–7.

[11] Penney g, Mair G, Pearson DWM. Outcomes of pregnancies in women with type 1 diabetes in Scotland: a national population-based study. Br J Obstet Gynaecol 2003;110:315–8.

[12] Casson IF, Clarke CA, Howard CV, et al. Outcomes in pregnancy in insulin dependent diabetic women: results of a five year population cohort study. Br Med J 1997;315:275–8.

[13] Macintosh MCM, Fleming KM, Bailey JA, et al. Perinatal mortality and congenital anomalies in babies of women with type 1 and type 2 diabetes in England, Wales, and Northern Ireland: population based study. Br Med J 2006;333:177.

[14] Mondestin MAJ, Ananth CV, Smulian JC, et al. Birth weight and fetal death in the United States: the effect of maternal diabetes during pregnancy. Am J Obstet Gynecol 2002;187: 922–6.

[15] Cundy T, Gamble G, Townend K, et al. Perinatal mortality in type 2 diabetes mellitus. Diabet Med 2000;17:33–9.

[16] Clausen TD, Mathiesen E, Ekbom P, et al. Poor pregnancy outcome in women with type 2 diabetes. Diabetes Care 2005;28:323–8.

[17] Dunne F, Brydon P, Smith K, et al. Pregnancy in women with type 2 diabetes: 12 years outcome data 1990–2002. Diabet Med 2003;20:734–8.

[18] O'Sullivan JB, Charles D, Mahan CM, et al. Gestational diabetes and perinatal mortality rate. Am J Obstet Gynecol 1973;116:901–4.

[19] White BM, Beischer NA. Perinatal mortality in the infants of diabetic women. Aust N Z J Obstet Gynaecol 1990;30:323–6.

[20] Beisher NA, Wein P, Sheedy MT, et al. Identification and treatment of women with hyperglycemia diagnosed during pregnancy can significantly reduce perinatal mortality rates. Aust N Z J Obstet Gynaecol 1996;36:239–47.

[21] Aberg A, Rydhstrom H, Kallen B, et al. Impaired glucose tolerance during pregnancy is associated with increased fetal mortality in preceding sibs. Acta Obstet Gynecol Scand 1997;76:212–7.

[22] Wood SL, Jick H, Sauve R. The risk of stillbirth in pregnancies before and after the onset of diabetes. Diabet Med 2003;20:703–7.

[23] Girz BA, Divon MY, Merkatz IR. Sudden fetal death in women with well-controlled, intensively monitored gestational diabetes. J Perinatol 1992;12:229–33.

[24] Challis K, Melo A, Burgalho A, et al. Gestational diabetes mellitus and fetal death in Mozambique: an incident case-referent study. Acta Obstet Gynecol Scand 2002;81: 560–3.

[25] Langer O, Yogev Y, Most O, et al. Gestational diabetes: the consequences of not treating. Am J Obstet Gynecol 2005;192:989–97.

[26] Silver RM, Varner MW, Reddy U, et al. Work-up of stillbirth: a review of the evidence. Am J Obstet Gynecol 2007;156:133–44.

[27] Coustan DR. Perinatal morbidity and mortality. In: Reece EA, Coustand DR, editors. Diabetes mellitus in pregnancy: principles and practice. New York: Churchill Livingstone; 1988. p. 537–45.

[28] Datta S, Brown WU. Acid base status in diabetic mothers and their infants following general or spinal anesthesia for cesarean section. Anesthesiology 1977;47:272–6.

[29] Bradley RJ, Brudenell JM, Nicolaides KH. Fetal acidosis and hyperlacticaemia diagnosed by cordocentesis in pregnancies complicated by maternal diabetes mellitus. Diabet Med 1991;8:464–8.

[30] Phillips AF, Dubin JW, Matty PJ, et al. Arterial hypoxemia and hyperinsulinemia in the chronically hyperglycemic fetal lamb. Pediatr Res 1982;16:653–8.

[31] Myers RE. Brain damage due to asphyxia: mechanism of causation. J Perinat Med 1981;9: 78–86.

[32] Damasceno DC, Volpato GT, de Mattos Paranhos Calderon I. Cunha Rudge Mv. Oxidative stress and diabetes in pregnant rats. Anim Reprod Sci 2002;72:235–44.

[33] Wentzel P, Jansson L, Eriksson UJ. Diabetes in pregnancy: uterine blood flow and embryonic development in the rat. Pediatr Res 1995;38:598–606.

[34] Cederberg J, Siman CM, Eriksson UJ. Combined treatment with vitamin E experimental diabetic pregnancy. Pediatr Res 2001;49:755–62.

[35] Gareskog M, Cederberg J, Eriksson UJ, et al. Maternal diabetes in vivo and high glucose concentration in vitro increases apoptosis in rat embryos. Reprod Toxicol 2007;23:63–74.

[36] Poston L, Briley AL, Seed PT, et al. Vitamin C and vitamin E in pregnant women at risk for pre-eclampsia (VIP trial): randomized placebo-controlled trial. Lancet 2006;367:1145–54.

[37] Freeman HP, Chu KC. Determinants of cancer disparities: barriers to cancer screening, diagnosis, and treatment. Surg Oncol Clin N Am 2005;14:655–69.

[38] Temple RC, Aldridge VJ, Murphy HR. Prepregnancy care and pregnancy outcomes in women with type 1 diabetes. Diabetes Care 2006;29:1744–9.

[39] Johnstone FD, Lindsay RS, Steel J. Type 1 diabetes and pregnancy: trends in birth weight over 40 years at a single clinic. Obstet Gynecol 2006;107:1297–302.

[40] Langer O, Rodriquez DA, Xenakis EM, et al. Intensified versus conventional management of gestational diabetes. Am J Obstet Gynecol 1994;170:1036–46.

[41] Nielsen GL, Moller M, Sorensen HT. HbA1C in early diabetic pregnancy and pregnancy outcomes: a Danish population-based cohort study of 573 pregnancies in women with type 1 diabetes. Diabetes Care 2006;29:2612–6.

[42] Nielsen GL, Sorensen HT, Neilsen PH, et al. Glycosylated hemoglobin as predictor of adverse fetal outcome in type 1 diabetic pregnancies. Acta Diabetol 1997;34:217–22.

[43] Langer O, Conway DL, Berkus MD, et al. A comparison of glyburide and insulin in women with gestational diabetes mellitus. N Engl J Med 2000;343:1134–8.

[44] Kjos SL, Leung A, Henry OA, et al. Antepartum surveillance in diabetic pregnancies: predictors of fetal distress in labor. Am J Obstet Gynecol 1995;173:1532–9.

[45] Brecher A, Tharakan T, Williams A, et al. Perinatal mortality in diabetic patients undergoing antepartum fetal evaluation: a case-control study. J Matern Fetal Neonatal Med 2002;12:423–7.

[46] Landon MB, Vickers S. Fetal surveillance in pregnancy complicated by diabetes mellitus: is it necessary? J Matern Fetal Neonatal Med 2002;12:413–6.

[47] Yoon BH, Romero R, Roh CR, et al. Relationship between the fetal biophysical profile score, umbilical artery Doppler velocimetry, and fetal blood acid-base status determined by cordocentesis. Am J Obstet Gynecol 1993;169:1586–94.

[48] Reece EA, Hagav Z, Assimakopoulos E, et al. Diabetes mellitus in pregnancy and the assessment of umbilical artery waveforms using pulsed wave Doppler ultrasonography. J Ultrasound Med 1994;13:73–80.

[49] Bracero LA, Figueroa R, Byrne DW, et al. Comparison of umbilical Doppler velocimetry, nonstress testing, and biophysical profile in pregnancies complicated by diabetes. J Ultrasound Med 1996;15:301–8.

[50] Bracero LA, Haberman S, Byrne DW. Maternal glycemic control and umbilical artery Doppler velocimetry. J Matern Fetal Neonatal Med 2002;12:342–8.

[51] Wong SF, Chan FY, Cincotta RB, et al. Use of umbilical artery Doppler velocimetry in the monitoring of pregnancy in women with pre-existing diabetes. Aust N Z J Obstet Gynaecol 2003;43:302–6.

[52] Fetal Macrosomia. American College of Obstetricians and Gynecologists Practice Bulletin 2000;22.

[53] Conway DL, Langer O. Elective delivery of infants with macrosomia in diabetic women: reduced shoulder dystocia versus increased cesarean deliveries. Am J Obstet Gynecol 1998;178:922–5.

[54] Alfirevic Z, Devane D, Gyte GM Continuous cardiotography (CTG) as a form of electronic fetal monitoring for fetal assessment during labor. Cochrane Database Syst Rev 2006;3:CD006066.

ELSEVIER
SAUNDERS

Obstet Gynecol Clin N Am
34 (2007) 309–322

OBSTETRICS AND
GYNECOLOGY
CLINICS
OF NORTH AMERICA

# Detection and Prevention of Macrosomia

## Andrea L. Campaigne, MD[a],
## Deborah L. Conway, MD[b],*

[a]Department of Obstetrics and Gynecology, The University of Texas Health Science Center
at San Antonio, 7703 Floyd Curl Drive, San Antonio, TX 78229, USA
[b]Department of Obstetrics and Gynecology, Division of Maternal-Fetal Medicine,
The University of Texas Health Science Center at San Antonio, 7703 Floyd Curl Drive,
San Antonio, TX 78229, USA

Definitions of excessive fetal growth generally employ a particular estimated or real birth weight "limit" regardless of gestational age, usually 4000 g or 4500 g. The usefulness of this definition is limited by not taking into account the factor of gestational age. For example, is a 4000-g infant at 36 weeks more vital to detect than a postterm macrosomic infant? With regard to assessing fetal growth in the diabetic pregnancy, many have turned instead to the definitions of large- and small-for-gestational-age (LGA and SGA, respectively) as more relevant standards for treatment and management because they take into account gestational age and better reflect deviations from the expected norm. Notwithstanding the variations in definitions, adverse outcome data for diabetic pregnancies complicated by excessive fetal growth are real. Associated perinatal and maternal morbidity include shoulder dystocia; brachial plexus injury; labor dystocia and operative delivery; and neonatal complications such as hypoglycemia, hyperbilirubinemia, intensive care admissions, and even perinatal mortality. Knowing these complications can occur, the authors are compelled to accurately identify the fetus/neonate at highest risk, and intervene appropriately to avoid the scenario. The question is then begged: How can we best predict adverse outcomes related to excessive fetal growth that can only truly be discovered at or *after* delivery?

The detection of excessive fetal growth is wrought with further challenges; the questions asked are layered with complexities.

---

* Corresponding author.
 *E-mail address:* conway@uthscsa.edu (D.L. Conway).

- To what *end* do we seek to detect excessive fetal growth? If only for de-livery management decisions, then an accurate near-term assessment is needed. On the other hand, detection of fetal overgrowth earlier in ges-tation would offer us the opportunity to impact the abnormal growth rate. Can and should the growth rate be "corrected" through changes in diabetic management?
- Is there an optimum method for estimating fetal weight in diabetics—by ultrasound, clinical maneuvers, or maternal perception—and how reli-able are our available methods? Are they equally reliable across the third trimester? Some limitations include the inaccuracy of ultrasound itself at extremes of birth weight; the multitude of formulae, thresholds, stan-dards, and definitions guiding our assessments; and the problem of latency, or scan-to-delivery interval.
- And, finally, is birth weight really the whole story? Or is detection of fetal "fatness" and/or disproportionate growth perhaps a more impor-tant finding, especially given the paradoxical finding that a large propor-tion of birth trauma and shoulder dystocia still occurs with birth weights *below* 4000 g? [1].

For the purpose of this review, studies focusing on pregnancies compli-cated by diabetes were selected whenever possible.

### Early detection and implications for treatment/prevention

At what point in gestation should we attempt to detect overgrowth? When does it start, and does that correlate to when it can be detected? What are the limitations of our ability to detect it? Can it be altered once detected, or is it biologically/physiologically programmed in the course of diabetes in pregnancy? Are the antenatal implications as critical as the peri-partum ones? In other words, does it matter if a diabetic mother has an in-fant that appears in early- to mid-gestation to be ahead of the growth curves for norms of gestational age?

A recent study by Holcomb and colleagues [2] sought to build on earlier studies [3–5] that first established fetal abdominal circumference (AC) "overgrowth" as a representation of accelerated somatic growth in diabetic pregnancies and a predictor for increased birth weight. Using a single ultra-sound examination at 28 to 32 weeks, they compared the performance of AC alone versus estimated fetal weight (EFW) to predict term birth weight greater than 90th percentile in an all-diabetic population (diet-controlled gestational diabetes mellitus [GDM] to insulin-treated pregestational diabe-tes mellitus). They evaluated LGA definitions by the Brenner standard ver-sus the California-based Williams standard. They concluded that AC performed as well as EFW, but that, as previously discovered, ultrasound prediction of excessive fetal growth yields significantly better negative than positive predictions (overall results: 89% sensitivity, 76% specificity,

50% positive predictive value, and 96% negative predictive value). Limitations of this study include that little information is given regarding the quality of glycemic control between scan and delivery as well as the small size of the study group (n = 84).

But what is the argument for using an early third-trimester ultrasound to detect excessive fetal growth and changing treatment to affect better diabetic control? Can doing so change the perinatal outcomes we are striving to avoid? Obviously, *not* treating is not an option, especially when abnormal fetal growth patterns are recognized. A large (n = 2775) retrospective cohort analysis [6] of uncontrolled GDM versus well-controlled GDM versus non-diabetic patients in 2005 demonstrated significantly higher rates of macrosomia (17% versus 7% versus 8%, respectively), LGA (29% versus 11% versus 11%), ponderal index (22% versus 13% versus 14%), shoulder dystocia (2.5% versus 0.9% versus 0.6%), and stillbirth (5.4/1000 versus 3.6/1000 versus 1.8/1000) in women who had uncontrolled GDM. The overall composite outcome index statistic (including many of those previously mentioned) was perhaps most telling, with at least one adverse outcome occurring in 59% of untreated versus 18% of treated and 11% of nondiabetic women. A randomized controlled trial of the same year (n = 1000 women who had "mild" GDM by oral glucose tolerance test results) [7], confirmed these retrospective data. Comparing an intervention group to a "routine care" or untreated group, significantly higher rates of macrosomia (21% versus 10), LGA (22% versus 13), shoulder dystocia (3% versus 1, $P = .07$), and stillbirth (not significant at three total events compared with 0, $P = .25$) were seen in the routine care group. It is clear that treatment matters in preventing excessive fetal growth in pregnancy complicated by diabetes.

The role ultrasound detection should play in directing diabetic treatment is less clear. Macrosomia rates in diabetic pregnancies may be higher than in the nondiabetic population despite excellent glycemic control, due to comorbidities and risk factors such as maternal obesity, maternal age, ethnicity, and weight gain during pregnancy. In addition, strict mid- to late-gestation glucose control has a known complication of *undergrowth*, or SGA. Raychaudhuri and Maresh [8] sought to elucidate if the poor correlation between blood glucose concentration and birth weight might be related to the gestational age at which control was achieved. Evaluating 76 consecutive insulin-dependent diabetic pregnant women, they sought to determine the timing of fetal growth acceleration by serial ultrasounds at 20, 24, 28, 32, and 34 weeks of completed gestation. In addition, data on the degree of glucose control were collected in the form of monthly glycosylated hemoglobin levels and mean capillary blood glucose values from home meter use. They compared the pregnancies in which the infant was LGA at birth (41% of their cohort) to the group delivering an average for gestational age (AGA) infant (51% of the cohort). Their data suggested that AC growth acceleration in the LGA group started at 20 to 24 weeks, but that the glycosylated hemoglobin showed significant differences (higher in the LGA group versus AGA) *before* the ultrasound findings were detectable (by 18 weeks). This led them to conclude that perhaps fetal growth acceleration was determined in the first half of pregnancy and may be continued to some degree despite improvements in diabetic control. These findings corroborate those of Keller and colleagues [9]. Evaluating 52 pregestational insulin-dependent diabetic pregnancies, they found evidence that accelerated AC growth before 24 weeks predicted macrosomia despite similarly tight glucose control over the weeks following the ultrasound estimation of fetal size.

A different result was found by Schaefer-Graf and colleagues [10] in 2004. Again using serial (monthly) ultrasounds at 20, 24, 28, 32, and 36 weeks gestation, they randomized women who had GDM to standard care (n = 100) versus ultrasound-directed therapy (n = 99). Level of glycemic control was used to determine need for initiation of insulin in the standard care group, based on fairly rigorous thresholds. In the ultrasound group, although routine self-monitoring of blood glucose was performed by the patients, the sole criterion for initiation of insulin therapy was a marker of excessive fetal growth (AC greater than 75th percentile). Thereafter, the ultrasound group was actually held to tighter glycemic targets than the standard group, an attempt to "correct" the excessive fetal growth. Rates of insulin initiation were similar between the two groups: 27.0% in the standard group and 36.4% in the ultrasound group. There were no significant differences among the outcomes considered (birth weight, LGA/SGA, neonatal body composition, neonatal hypoglycemia, neonatal ICU admissions, or cesarean section delivery rate) and LGA rates in both groups were comparable to a nondiabetic population. The authors concluded that management based on fetal growth characteristics provided similar perinatal outcomes as traditional management strategies based on glucose monitoring, perhaps providing an alternative management strategy for milder cases of gestational diabetes.

Buchanan and colleagues [11] evaluated the concept of ultrasound detection of the fetus most "at risk" for excessive growth, combined with the tailoring of medical therapy to reverse it. Using a single early third-trimester ultrasound (between 29–33 weeks) to guide treatment of GDM, they compared four study groups: a "low-risk" population (GDM with fetal AC < 75th percentile) who received standard diet therapy (n = 171); high-risk, refused randomization (GDM with fetal AC ≥ 75th percentile) who also received no more than standard diet therapy (n = 24); and two other high-risk groups who were randomized to diet alone (n = 29) versus empiric insulin therapy (n = 30). Results revealed LGA rates of 14%, 38%, 45%, and 13%, respectively. Important conclusions from this evidence are that a single fetal ultrasound criterion can be used to risk stratify patients who have GDM for the outcome of macrosomia as well as that insulin lowered the LGA rate in pregnancies identified by this single fetal ultrasound characteristic. Others have sought to further characterize fetal abdominal measurements alone for their ability to predict macrosomia with varying degrees of success [12,13].

### Detection—is ultrasound better than physician or maternal perception?

According to the American College of Obstetricians and Gynecologists (ACOG) Practice Bulletin on macrosomia [14], methods that aid the clinician in detecting/predicting macrosomia include assessment of maternal risk factors, ultrasound measurement, and clinical appraisal—both by physician examination and maternal estimation. Chauhan and colleagues [15] in 1992 published a comparison of fetal weight estimation by maternal perception (including only multiparous women) versus clinical (ie, Leopold maneuvers) and sonographic means (n = 106). The results demonstrated the comparability of maternal judgment to the physician's best tools. Maternal estimates were found to be within 10% of actual birth weight 70% of the time, compared with 66% of clinical estimates and only 42% of sonographic estimates. In addition, the mean error in grams and accordingly the mean percent error were both less for maternal versus clinical and sonographic (305 g [8.7%] versus 314 g [9.0%] versus 564 g [15.6%], respectively). This study seems to validate maternal perception as a reliable estimate of birth weight. Limitations of this method include the requirement of patients' parity and a lack of data on the reliability at extremes of birth weight (eg, macrosomia) or on data specific to pregnancies complicated by diabetes.

Although the latter study seems to underestimate the accuracy of sonographic EFW, it does highlight the potential place for physician clinical estimates, a part of the art of obstetrics previously thought to be notoriously scientifically irreproducible (with reported sensitivities ranging from 24%-97% and with specificities from 98%–82%). In a review of sonographic versus clinical methods in diagnosing macrosomia, O'Reilly-Green and Divon [16] found the accuracy of both measures to be comparable to one another and more reproducible in the pooled literature, with 67% of clinical estimates and 66% of sonographic estimates within 10% of actual birth weight. This review also separately evaluated the sensitivity of both methods when actual birth weight exceeded 4000 g. Pooled analysis found proportions dropped to 58% for clinical and 51% for sonographic estimates within 10% of actual birth weight under these circumstances, with mean absolute error of 245 g and 500 g, respectively. This illustrates the decreasing sensitivity/accuracy of all commonly used methods of fetal weight estimation, at macrosomic-range birth weights.

To address the particular problem of fetal weight estimation in the pregnancies at highest risk for excessive fetal growth, several studies have focused on a diabetic population specifically. Hendrix and colleagues [17] found clinical estimates to have significantly better mean standardized absolute error and percentage of estimates within 10% of actual birth weight than ultrasound estimates at birth weights of at least 4000 g but not at birth weights less than 4000 g. Johnstone and colleagues [18] compared clinical versus sonographic estimation in their ability to predict macrosomia,

performing serial scans at 28 weeks gestation, 34 weeks gestation, and before delivery. They found that the performance of clinical measurement
in prediction of macrosomia increases with increasing gestational age, but
that it performs as well as ultrasound measurements at term.

Hirata and colleagues [19] studied only fetuses clinically estimated to be
at least 3900 g by Leopold maneuvers in early labor (21% diabetic) and
compared the performance of different ultrasound formulae in predicting
macrosomic-range birth weight. They compared the formulae of Shepard,
Hadlock 1–4, and Tamura, as well as original formulations, and found
the best performing formulae to be ones that used AC and femur length
(FL) to the exclusion of head circumference/biparietal diameter (HC/
BPD) in the highly-restricted macrosomic population. The authors highlighted the concern that in studying a variable of limited prevalence (ie, macrosomia) in a population with specific risk factors (diabetes in pregnancy),
perhaps it is neither possible nor wise to apply standards that have been developed for the general population.

### Detection—ultrasound accuracy

In spite of the lack of proof that the use of ultrasound to estimate fetal
weight in the diabetic pregnancy is superior to other methods of fetal
weight estimation, it is still widely used in day-to-day clinical practice.
Factors contributing to reliance on ultrasound are its broad availability,
ease and speed in obtaining results, and perceived objectivity as an assessment technique. How dependable is it, and what are its limitations? A pioneering systematic review [20] was recently undertaken to judge the
accuracy of ultrasound biometry in predicting macrosomia. The comprehensive data included over 19,000 women, 16 formulae for EFW (including typical biometrics), and four criteria for AC thresholds. As such, one
of the unique weaknesses in this study represents a weakness experienced
daily by physicians in ultrasound estimation—extensive heterogeneity in
methods as well as in reference thresholds. The data were assessed by summary receiver operating characteristic curves and the accuracy of each
method evaluated by summary likelihood ratios, which signified, according
to the authors, "by how much a given ultrasound test result raises or
lowers the probability of having a macrosomic newborn." Both categories
(EFW and AC) yielded pooled likelihood ratios (high LR+ compared with
LR−), indicating that formulae across the board are more accurate at ruling in macrosomia than at ruling it out, a conclusion contrary to some
aforementioned individual studies. In addition, when formulae for composite EFW were compared head-to-head against those using AC alone,
analysis indicated similar overall accuracies. Given the lack of precision,
though, the authors could not identify one formula worthy of recommendation over any other. The primary shortcoming of this study for the

purposes of this review, however, is that the presence or contribution of diabetes is not addressed.

One year prior, a review article evaluated in similar fashion the current state of our ability to detect macrosomia, in an effort to develop an algorithm for treatment/management once detected. Chauhan and colleagues [21] compared 20 articles (representing nearly 8800 patients, 80% from the United States) using various formulae for calculating ultrasound EFW with various ultrasound-to-delivery intervals. Furthermore, they subanalyzed data relating to diabetic and postterm patients as risk factors for macrosomia unique from the routine general obstetric population. The subset of articles representing the sonographic detection of macrosomia in the diabetic population included three articles and 442 patients. The authors found wide disparity among the macrosomia incidence rates reported in the general obstetric population (3%–55%) and again noted wide ranges of sensitivities and specificities among their ultrasound detection methods, with posttest probabilities of 15%–79%. However, they noted that unlike the general obstetric population, the literature on sonographic detection of macrosomia among diabetic patients was fairly consistent, with macrosomia rates of 19%–26%, sensitivities of 33%–69%, specificities of 77%–98%, and yielding posttest probabilities of 44%–81%.

### Detection—timing and adjustments

The concept of latency, or scan-to-delivery interval, must also be considered as the authors analyze the accuracy and reliability of fetal weight estimation by ultrasound in the care of a pregnant woman who has diabetes. With the potential inaccuracy of ultrasound established, how does one extrapolate data obtained remotely to predict impact on delivery? This issue has been handled in a multitude of ways, certainly not standardized across the literature.

In addition, many have pointed out features that compromise the quality (and therefore the accuracy) of ultrasound biometry at term including descent of the fetal head into the pelvis, decreasing amniotic fluid volume, and maternal body weight/habitus. How have investigators handled these variables? Do we have evidence to support a generally accepted time frame for near-term ultrasound evaluation or a manner of adjusting our routine or early third-trimester evaluations?

The most apparent conclusion is no, given the wide range of latency between ultrasound estimation of fetal weight and delivery. For example, in Chauhan's aforementioned review [21], latency varied from 3 days to more than 23 days. Some have suggested a gestational-age associated projection or adjustment (in grams per day or grams per week) to account for the delay between prediction and outcome (delivery). Some examples of the available evidence are summarized in Table 1 [22–25].

Table 1
Effect of latency and formulae on calculation of EFW

| Authors | Study size | Diabetic status/proportion | Macrosomia rate | Latency (Scan-to-delivery interval) | U/S EFW formula/ae applied | Results |
|---|---|---|---|---|---|---|
| Farrell et al [22] | N = 164 | 100% DM (32% PGDM, 68% GDM) | 26% | U/S within 10 d of delivery | Hadlock, Shepard, Vintzileos, and Campbell & Wilkin 25 g/d adjusted weight gain over scan-to-delivery interval applied | Hadlock and Shepard tended to underestimate; Vintzileos and C&W tended to overestimate; for infants with BW >4 kg, C&W generated smallest range between limits of agreement; 68% of estimated weights were within 10% of actual BW using the AC only formula (C&W) |
| Sokol et al [23] | N = 4831 | 3% DM (?PGDM versus GDM) | 16.9% DM 6.4% general | U/S within 14 d of delivery | Hadlock (standard) versus formula adjusted for DM status and maternal weight and height no fixed growth rate, cubic growth model based on U/S EFW | AC, FL, and HC each regressed on BW to obtain EFW based on each variable; significantly increased risk for BW >4 kg when EFW based on AC is larger than that based on FL or HC |

| | N | DM status | | Days | Method | Comments |
|---|---|---|---|---|---|---|
| Best and Pressman [24] | N = 1823 | 7.3% DM (PGDM versus GDM) | 23.3% DM 9.2% general | Avg 19.4 d DM avg 23.4 d general (ie, ~34–37 wk) | Brenner (standard) versus gestation-adjusted projection method | Prediction of BW using the gestation-adjusted projection method is at least as accurate in diabetic patients as in controls |
| Rosati et al [25] | N = 732 | No comment on DM status | 14% LGA | 7 d | Original gestational-age specific model versus Hadlock, Shepard, C&W, and others | AC and AD show the highest sensitivity of all parameters in identifying macrosomia, but EFW offers highest PPV (90%) and accuracy (94%) |

*Abbreviations:* AD, abdominal diameter; BW, birth weight; C&W, Campbell & Wilkin; HC, head circumference; PGDM, pregestational diabetes mellitus; PPV, positive predictive value; U/S, ultrasound.

### Detection—altered fetal growth and new ultrasound horizons

As acknowledged in the ACOG Practice Bulletin [14] on the subject, "Macrosomia produced by maternal glucose intolerance is different from that associated with other predisposing factors." Citing anthropometric studies evaluating neonatal body composition of macrosomic newborns of diabetic versus nondiabetic mothers, increased truncal and upper extremity adiposity was established. Increasingly, then, ultrasound diagnosis of macrosomia has turned to new techniques for evaluating fetal fat distribution as a surrogate for, or in addition to, simple estimation of fetal weight in assessing risk of macrosomia and its sequelae.

Landon and colleagues [26] as early as 1991 identified humeral soft tissue thickness as a promising tool. In a small study of diabetic pregnancies, the authors concluded that humeral soft tissue thickness may distinguish large-for-gestational-age fetuses with such abnormal body composition as more at risk of birth injury at delivery than symmetrically large fetuses. In another small study comparing diabetic (GDM and pre-GDM) versus nondiabetic pregnancies, Sood and colleagues [27] evaluated humeral soft tissue thickness in a population selected to be at risk for macrosomia. Participants all had at least one of the following risk factors for macrosomia: fundal height 3 cm greater than gestational age, GDM, pre-GDM, or a previous delivery of a macrosomic infant. Of their cohort, based on the above risk profiling, they had a surprising 55% macrosomia rate ($>4000$ g), a 57% cesarean delivery rate, and an over 6% shoulder dystocia rate. They found humeral soft tissue thickness to be significantly higher in macrosomic fetuses, without apparent effect of maternal diabetic status. When compared with sonographic estimated fetal weight, the authors found humeral soft tissue thickness to be more sensitive (88% versus 71%) but less specific (75% versus 91%) in predicting macrosomia.

In 1992, Hill and colleagues [28] studied subcutaneous soft tissue thickness measurements at three other discreet locations—midcalf, midthigh, and abdominal circumference—throughout gestation (15–42 weeks) on controls versus fetuses at both extremes of abnormal growth (SGA and LGA). They concluded that because of the degree in overlap of measurements between groups, neither growth retardation nor macrosomia could be reliably predicted by their methods. No diabetic patients were included as either controls or in the LGA group. In contrast, an Italian study published in 2003 by Larciprete and colleagues [29] sought to establish reference values for fetal subcutaneous tissue thickness throughout gestation for a "healthy" population versus a well-controlled GDM population (pre-GDM was excluded). The standard therapy and glucose targets for the GDM arm were explicitly well established. Subcutaneous tissue thickness was assessed serially at four locations: midarm, midthigh, abdomen, and subscapular. Although mean birth weight for the two groups (healthy versus GDM) is reported, there is no indication of the macrosomia rate. However, they found significant differences in fetal fat mass values at all four locations near term (35+ weeks) even in well-controlled gestational diabetes.

Another tool for appraisal of abnormal fetal fat distribution in pregnancies complicated by macrosomia is the cheek-to-cheek diameter (CCD), primarily reported by Abramowicz and colleagues. In 1993 [30], they found CCD to be significantly less in SGA fetuses and significantly greater in LGA fetuses than in AGA fetuses. In addition, they reported that LGA fetuses of diabetic mothers had an increased CCD/BPD ratio, which they concluded permitted insight into the possible mechanism underlying macrosomia in this population. In another study in 1997 [31], Abramowicz and colleagues sought to combine CCD with BPD and AC to produce a new formula for ultrasound estimation of fetal weight. They found incorporating CCD into an estimated fetal weight formula increased the proportion of estimates within 10% of actual birth weight from 73% (by BPD/AC alone formula) to over 95% when CCD was incorporated. However, they also noted that CCD did not significantly improve fetal weight prediction in nonmacrosomic fetuses, concluding that perhaps CCD explains more of the variance in birth weight than other parameters.

Evaluation of the "fatness" of the diabetic fetus has been taken even to the extreme of assessment of enlargement of the cardiac interventricular septum [32]. The horizon for the antenatal measurement of the adiposity of the diabetic fetus appears to be in new volumetric techniques, including three-dimensional ultrasound [33,35,38] and MRI [34,36,37,41].

## Closing statements

Even in light of an outcome such as macrosomia, which universally affects obstetricians, how can we begin to agree on a strategy to target prevention of macrosomia by way of diabetic control when there is so little consensus on gestational diabetes—from screening and diagnosis to treatment and antenatal monitoring? In addition, there is confusing evidence. Several early studies demonstrated reduction in macrosomia and LGA rates with tight glucose control. However, others have highlighted the fact that even despite tight glucose control, diabetic patients can and do produce macrosomic fetuses and abnormal neonatal body compositions that put them at risk for shoulder dystocia and its complications, perhaps as a result of other risk factors, such as obesity. In addition, studies have also highlighted a further concern—that in the presence of the lowest average mean glucose thresholds, growth can actually be compromised by the strictest diabetic control, with SGA rates increasing even in diabetic patients when mean blood glucose is held to below "normal" or 86 mg/dL. Additionally, what then should be used to guide decisions about when and how to treat—blood glucose self-monitoring values or ultrasound assessment?

As stated in the ACOG Practice Bulletin on Gestational Diabetes [39], "The first consideration in selecting a therapy for GDM is a determination of the treatment goals." Clearly, gestational and pregestational diabetes and even simply maternal glycemia or impaired glucose tolerance have wide-ranging impact on pregnancy outcomes from beginning to end; from conception to delivery; and beyond, for both the woman and her offspring. To this end, Langer has suggested [40] that we think of glucose control as a continuum, with targets "flexible" to meet the goals at hand. For example, pregestationally and in the first trimester, one set of "norms" or targets may be considered to prevent early outcomes such as spontaneous abortion or congenital malformations. Macrosomia is only one such variable, with concern focused primarily on interventions in mid-to-late gestation to impact the phase of the most rapid fetal growth. It is overly simplistic to try to identify optimal glycemic thresholds, fetal growth characteristics, and methods of detection in the prevention of fetal overgrowth and its attendant morbidities that can be applied to all pregnancies. We can only hope that, as our understanding of the pathophysiology of diabetes in pregnancy grows, we can "fine-tune" our therapy and surveillance to meet the needs of an individual woman who has diabetes and her fetus.

# References

[1] Gonen R, Spiegel D, Abend M. Is macrosomia predictable, and are shoulder dystocia and birth trauma preventable? Obstet Gynecol 1996;88:526–9.
[2] Holcomb WL Jr, Mostello DJ, Gray DL. Abdominal circumference vs. estimated weight to predict large for gestational age birth weight in diabetic pregnancy. Clin Imaging 2000;24:1–7.
[3] Ogata ES, Sabbagha R, Metzger BE, et al. Serial ultrasonography to assess evolving fetal macrosomia: studies in 23 pregnant diabetic women. JAMA 1980;243:2405–8.
[4] Bochner CJ, Medearis AL, Williams J 3rd, et al. Early third-trimester ultrasound screening in gestational diabetes to determine the risk of macrosomia and labor dystocia at term. Am J Obstet Gynecol 1987;157:703–8.
[5] Landon MB, Mintz MC, Gabbe SG. Sonographic evaluation of fetal abdominal growth: predictor of the large-for-gestational-age infant in pregnancies complicated by diabetes mellitus. Am J Obstet Gynecol 1989;160:115–21.
[6] Langer O, Yogev Y, Most O, et al. Gestational diabetes: the consequences of not treating. Am J Obstet Gynecol 2005;192:989–97.
[7] Crowther CA, Hiller JE, Moss JR, et al. Effect of treatment of gestational diabetes mellitus on pregnancy outcomes. N Engl J Med 2005;352:2477–86.
[8] Raychaudhuri K, Maresh MJ. Glycemic control throughout pregnancy and fetal growth in insulin-dependent diabetes. Obstet Gynecol 2000;95:190–4.
[9] Keller JD, Metzger BE, Dooley SL, et al. Infants of diabetic mothers with accelerated fetal growth by ultrasonography: are they all alike? Am J Obstet Gynecol 1990;163:893–7.
[10] Schaefer-Graf UM, Kjos SL, Fauzan OH, et al. A randomized trial evaluating a predominantly fetal growth-based strategy to guide management of gestational diabetes in caucasian women. Diabetes Care 2004;27:297–302.
[11] Buchanan TA, Kjos SL, Montoro MN, et al. Use of fetal ultrasound to select metabolic therapy for pregnancies complicated by mild gestational diabetes. Diabetes Care 1994;17:275–83.

[12] Gilby JR, Williams MC, Spellacy WN. Fetal abdominal circumference measurements of 35 and 38 cm as predictors of macrosomia. A risk factor for shoulder dystocia. J Reprod Med 2000;45:936–8.

[13] Henrichs C, Magann EF, Brantley KL, et al. Detecting fetal macrosomia with abdominal circumference alone. J Reprod Med 2003;48:339–42.

[14] American College of Obstetricians and Gynecologists, ACOG Practice Bulletin; Macrosomia.

[15] Chauhan SP, Lutton PM, Bailey KJ, et al. Intrapartum clinical, sonographic, and parous patients' estimates of newborn birth weight. Obstet Gynecol 1992;79:956–8.

[16] O'Reilly-Green C, Divon M. Sonographic and clinical methods in the diagnosis of macrosomia. Clin Obstet Gynecol 2000;43:309–20.

[17] Hendrix NW, Morrison JC, McLaren RA, et al. Clinical and sonographic estimates of birth weight among diabetic parturients. J Matern Fetal Investig 1998;8:17–20.

[18] Johnstone FD, Prescott RJ, Steel JM, et al. Clinical and ultrasound prediction of macrosomia in diabetic pregnancy. Br J Obstet Gynaecol 1996;103:747–54.

[19] Hirata GI, Medearis AL, Horenstein J, et al. Ultrasonographic estimation of fetal weight in the clinically macrosomic fetus. Am J Obstet Gynecol 1990;162:238–42.

[20] Coomarasamy A, Connock M, Thornton J, et al. Accuracy of ultrasound biometry in the prediction of macrosomia: a systematic quantitative review. BJOG 2005;112:1461–6.

[21] Chauhan SP, Grobman WA, Gherman RA, et al. Suspicion and treatment of the macrosomic fetus: a review. Am J Obstet Gynecol 2005;193:332–46.

[22] Farrell T, Fraser R, Chan K. Ultrasonic fetal weight estimation in women with pregnancy complicated by diabetes. Acta Obstet Gynecol Scand 2004;83:1065–6.

[23] Sokol RJ, Chik L, Dombrowski MP, et al. Correctly identifying the macrosomic fetus: improving ultrasonography-based prediction. Am J Obstet Gynecol 2000;182:1489–95.

[24] Best G, Pressman EK. Ultrasonographic prediction of birth weight in diabetic pregnancies. Obstet Gynecol 2002;99:740–4.

[25] Rosati P, Exacoustos C, Caruso A, et al. Ultrasound diagnosis of fetal macrosomia. Ultrasound Obstet Gynecol 1992;2:23–9.

[26] Landon MB, Sonek J, Foy P, et al. Sonographic measurement of fetal humeral soft tissue thickness in pregnancy complicated by GDM. Diabetes 1991;40(Suppl2):66–70.

[27] Sood AK, Yancey M, Richards D. Prediction of fetal macrosomia using humeral soft tissue thickness. Obstet Gynecol 1995;85:937–40.

[28] Hill LM, Guzick D, Boyles D, et al. Subcutaneous tissue thickness cannot be used to distinguish abnormalities of fetal growth. Obstet Gynecol 1992;80:268–71.

[29] Larciprete G, Valensise H, Vasapollo B, et al. Fetal subcutaneous tissue thickness (SCTT) in healthy and gestational diabetic pregnancies. Ultrasound Obstet Gynecol 2003;22:591–7.

[30] Abramowicz JS, Sherer DM, Woods JR Jr. Ultrasonographic measurement of cheek-to-cheek diameter in fetal growth disturbances. Am J Obstet Gynecol 1993;169:405–8.

[31] Abramowicz JS, Robischon K, Cox C. Incorporating sonographic cheek-to-cheek diameter, biparietal diameter and abdominal circumference improves weight estimation in the macrosomic fetus. Ultrasound Obstet Gynecol 1997;9:409–13.

[32] Bethune M, Bell R. Evaluation of the measurement of the fetal fat layer, interventricular septum and abdominal circumference percentile in the prediction of macrosomia in pregnancies affected by gestational diabetes. Ultrasound Obstet Gynecol 2003;22:586–90.

[33] Chang FM, Liang RI, Ko HC, et al. Three-dimensional ultrasound-assessed fetal thigh volumetry in predicting birth weight. Obstet Gynecol 1997;90:331–9.

[34] Uotila J, Dastidar P, Heinonen T, et al. Magnetic resonance imaging compared to ultrasonography in fetal weight and volume estimation in diabetic and normal pregnancy. Acta Obstet Gynecol Scand 2000;79:255–9.

[35] Schild RL, Fimmers R, Hansmann M. Fetal weight estimation by three-dimensional ultrasound. Ultrasound Obstet Gynecol 2000;16:445–52.

[36] Tukeva TA, Salmi H, Poutanen VP, et al. Fetal shoulder measurements by fast and ultrafast MRI techniques. J Magn Reson Imaging 2001;13:938–42.

[37] Hassibi S, Farhataziz N, Zaretsky M, et al. Optimization of fetal weight estimates using MRI: comparison of acquisitions. AJR Am J Roentgenol 2004;183:487–92.

[38] Lee W, Deter RL, Ebersole JD, et al. Birth weight prediction by three-dimensional ultrasonography: fractional limb volume. J Ultrasound Med 2001;20:1283–92.

[39] American College of Obstetricians and Gynecologists. ACOG practice bulletin: gestational diabetes. Obstet Gynecol 2001;98:525–38.

[40] Langer O. A spectrum of glucose thresholds may effectively prevent complications in the pregnant diabetic patient. Semin Perinatol 2002;26:196–205.

[41] American Diabetes Association. Gestational diabetes mellitus. Diabetes Care 2004;27(Suppl 1): S88–90.

ELSEVIER
SAUNDERS

Obstet Gynecol Clin N Am
34 (2007) 323–334

OBSTETRICS AND
GYNECOLOGY
CLINICS
OF NORTH AMERICA

# Labor and Delivery Management for Women With Diabetes

## J. Seth Hawkins, MD, Brian M. Casey, MD*

*Department of Obstetrics and Gynecology, University of Texas Southwestern Medical Center,
5323 Harry Hines Boulevard, Dallas, Texas 75390, USA*

More than 40 years ago, Dr. John B. O'Sullivan's [1] pioneering work on diabetes established that women with glucose intolerance during pregnancy are at increased risk of developing diabetes in the future. Subsequently, he reported that glucose intolerance identified during pregnancy also has important implications for the outcome of pregnancy. For instance, those women with milder forms of glucose intolerance seemed to be at risk for delivery of large infants and preeclampsia [2]. Since 1966, it has been reported that insulin therapy mitigates many of these associated complications and reduces the number of overgrown infants [3]. Several more recent prospective trials of insulin therapy in such women have also demonstrated a reduction in mean birth weight, but have not convincingly shown a reduction in the risk for cesarean delivery [4,5]. Conversely, some retrospective or nonrandomized studies have indicated that a reduction in cesarean delivery rate is possible through aggressive diabetes management [6,7]. These and many other investigators have advanced the understanding of diabetes during pregnancy and enabled obstetric providers to more safely deliver healthy babies to women with either preexisting or gestational diabetes [8–11].

Before arrival on labor and delivery by a pregnant woman with diabetes, there are a number of questions that an obstetric provider should consider. These include the following:

1. What are the obstetrical implications of diabetes?
2. What is the optimal timing of delivery?
3. When is it appropriate to perform a cesarean delivery?
4. How should blood glucose be managed during labor?

* Corresponding author.
*E-mail address:* brian.casey@utsouthwestern.edu (B.M. Casey).

Consideration of these factors is important to maximizing pregnancy outcome, particularly during the intrapartum period.

## Obstetrical implications of diabetes

Pregnancies complicated by diabetes are at risk for a number of adverse outcomes. Several of these outcomes directly affect the labor and delivery process and are linked to maternal age, duration of disease, and glycemic control during pregnancy. Briefly, these outcomes include fetal overgrowth, difficult delivery, preterm birth (often necessitated by supervening medical complications), hypertension, stillbirth, neonatal hypoglycemia, and admission to the neonatal intensive care unit.

As suggested above, the adverse perinatal outcomes associated with diabetes are influenced by the severity and duration of the glucose intolerance in a continuous fashion. Some of these outcomes are increased even in women with mild forms of glucose intolerance but without the diagnosis of gestational diabetes. For example, women with an increased 50-g glucose screen but a normal 100-g glucose tolerance test have been shown to be at increased risk for adverse obstetrical outcomes [12–15]. Similar findings have been reported in women with single abnormal values on a 75- or 100-g glucose tolerance test but without the diagnosis of diabetes [16–19]. Pregnancies complicated by more severe forms of diabetes, as in Type 1 and Type 2 diabetes mellitus, are at a progressively higher risk of adverse maternal and perinatal outcomes [20]. Moreover, women with poor glycemic control are at especially increased risk for pregnancy complications when compared with those with similar diabetes classification but with good glycemic control [21].

Apart from the severity of diabetes and glycemic control achieved during pregnancy, certain associated comorbidities also affect the risk of these pregnancy complications. The most common of these comorbidities is obesity. For example, obese women with gestational diabetes have a significantly increased risk of adverse outcomes when compared with those of normal weight. Specifically, obese women with gestational diabetes are 2 to 3 times more likely to deliver an overgrown infant [22]. A second common comorbidity of overt diabetes is chronic hypertension. Both chronic hypertension and diabetes are risk factors for preeclampsia, a diagnosis that commonly results in an indicated preterm birth.

### Fetal overgrowth

One of the primary concerns of the obstetric provider who attends the labor of a woman with diabetes is fetal size and the associated risk of a difficult delivery. In women with overt diabetes, fetal size can be excessive. However, in a woman with overt diabetes and evidence of vasculopathy, poor placental perfusion may paradoxically lead to delivery of a smaller, potentially growth-restricted baby [23]. The chief consequence of the diagnosis to women with gestational diabetes seems to be delivery of an overgrown infant [24].

Vaginal delivery of an overgrown baby is associated with a number of adverse outcomes for both mother and infant. The most feared of these outcomes is shoulder dystocia, identified when passage of the infant is obstructed by impaction of the fetal shoulder on the maternal pelvis, and the potential for fetal injury or asphyxiation. Neonatal risks of shoulder dystocia include clavicular or humeral fractures and brachial plexus injury [25–27]. A case series of 157 women with and without diabetes [26] who spontaneously delivered babies weighing at least 4500 g reported a shoulder dystocia rate of 18.5%. Erb palsy occurred in approximately 25% of the children whose delivery was complicated by shoulder dystocia. Clavicular fractures occurred in a similar proportion. Two of these infants whose deliveries were complicated by shoulder dystocia died. Obstetric providers recognize the following two relationships: first, diabetes is associated with larger infants, and second, the risk of shoulder dystocia increases with increasing birth weight [27]. Thus, many directly link diabetes with shoulder dystocia. This association is the driving force behind labor induction practice and recommendations for cesarean delivery in women with diabetes [28]. Importantly, however, only 12% to 15% of shoulder dystocia cases occur in women with diabetes [29,30]. Nevertheless, the risk of shoulder dystocia among women with diabetes during pregnancy, even after adjustment for maternal size, appears to be increased in women with either mild gestational diabetes [24] or overt diabetes [31].

Adverse maternal outcomes associated with difficult vaginal delivery include an increased risk of severe perineal laceration [26,32,33] and subsequent urinary and/or fecal incontinence [34]. Several studies have found operative delivery and episiotomy to be risk factors for pelvic floor dysfunction [34,35]. Importantly, operative vaginal delivery and fetal overgrowth are not the only risk factors for urinary incontinence. Familial predisposition is also a potent determinant of subsequent urinary incontinence [36]. Whether diabetes itself is associated with adverse urogynecological sequelae also remains to be determined. Interestingly, a large population-based study in Sweden reported that diabetes (either Type 1 or gestational) at the time of pregnancy was associated with a twofold increased risk for stress urinary incontinence surgery, even after stratification for episiotomy and birth weight [37].

*Preeclampsia*

Women with overt diabetes are at a significantly increased risk of developing preeclampsia, with the greatest risk identified in women with evidence of diabetic nephropathy (Table 1). O'Sullivan [2] first noted the relationship between gestational diabetes and preeclampsia. Subsequently, even women with mild glucose intolerance but without the diagnosis of gestational diabetes, have been shown to have at least some increased risk of hypertensive

Table 1
Risk of preeclampsia for women with overt diabetes by White classification

| White class | Garner (1995) [23] n = 117 | Sibai et al (2000) n = 462 |
|---|---|---|
| B | 5 of 46 (10.9%) | 17 of 157 (10.8%) |
| C | 8 of 61 (13.1%) | 42 of 191 (22.0%) |
| D, F, R | 3 of 10 (30%) | 33 of 114 (28.9%) |
| Overall | 16 of 117 (13.7%) | 92 of 462 (19.9%) |

disorders during pregnancy [12,16–19,38]. Similarly, the rate of hypertension in women with mild gestational diabetes is increased compared with the general obstetric population [24]. The risk of preeclampsia also seems to be influenced by duration of glucose intolerance. Indeed, women with mild gestational diabetes diagnosed early in pregnancy are more likely to be diagnosed with preeclampsia compared with women routinely diagnosed [39,40]. Moreover, the degree of glycemic control in those with gestational diabetes also appears to affect the risk of preeclampsia. Yogev and colleagues [41] reported that higher mean glucose values in women with gestational diabetes are associated with a twofold increased risk of preeclampsia.

*Stillbirth*

In women with overt diabetes, the risk of stillbirth is increased regardless of etiology (ie, Type 1 versus Type 2 diabetes) [42]. Recent studies describe a fetal death rate of 11 to 21 per 1000 for women with overt diabetes [43,44]. Women with gestational diabetes and fasting hyperglycemia or those with poor glycemic control also face an increased risk of stillbirth [8,9,21]. Conversely, women with mild, diet-treated gestational diabetes do not appear to be at increased risk of stillbirth [24]. Report of a large Canadian database of over 88,000 births weighing more than 500 g includes 709 stillbirths with a 97% autopsy rate. There was no increased risk of stillbirth in women with mild diet-treated diabetes, while women treated with insulin have a significantly higher fetal death rate [45]. In summary, stillbirth in pregnancy complicated by diabetes generally occurs in women with insulin-treated diabetes and poor glycemic control in the third trimester [23,46].

*Congenital malformations*

The pathophysiology of malformations in pregnancies complicated by diabetes is not well understood [47]; however, formation of free radicals and deficient expression of the Pax3 gene by an embryo exposed to hyperglycemia has been indicated as a possible mechanism [48,49]. Sheffield and colleagues [50] reported that common malformations in women with diabetes include those of the nervous system (neural tube defects, hydrocephaly, and microcephally), cardiovascular system (septal wall defects and hypoplastic heart), gastrointestinal system (ventral wall defects and intestinal atresia), and renal system (agenesis and dysplasia). The most significant risk factor for malformations in pregnancies complicated by diabetes is poor glycemic control during embryogenesis [51–53]. This risk is especially high in women with fasting hyperglycemia [50]. Improved glycemic control has been reported to be beneficial for reducing the risk of these malformations [21,54].

Congenital malformations in infants of women with diabetes may present complex obstetrical challenges. Challenges posed by these malformations include decisions regarding route of delivery and type of uterine incision. Fetuses with malformations may prompt consideration for cesarean delivery. For example, the optimal route of delivery for a fetus with a neural tube defect is controversial and, although cesarean delivery has not been shown to be uniformly beneficial, delivery at a tertiary center is recommended [55]. Other anomalies, such as ventral wall defects, may be delivered vaginally depending on the type and extent of the defect [56].

## The optimal timing of delivery

Several considerations govern timing of delivery. First, there is a need to balance the risks of stillbirth and iatrogenic preterm delivery. Second, the development of supervening maternal medical complications, such as severe preeclampsia, may necessitate early delivery. Third, there may be a need to also intervene for fetal well-being such as diminished fetal growth or abnormal antepartum fetal testing.

### Insulin-treated diabetes

In women whose pregnancies are complicated by insulin-treated diabetes, timing of delivery is primarily determined by the desire to avoid stillbirth. Intentional delivery of women with insulin-treated diabetes at 38 weeks gestation is intended to reduce the risk of stillbirth. This practice may increase cesarean delivery rates in these women and has prompted some to expectantly manage women with good glycemic control until 40 completed weeks of gestation. However, one study failed to detect a benefit to expectant management beyond 38 weeks of gestation as there was no decrease in cesarean delivery rates but rather an increase in large-for-gestational age infants and shoulder dystocia [57]. Similarly, Rayburn and colleagues [58] found that routine delivery at 38 weeks for women with insulin-treated diabetes was not associated with increased maternal or fetal intrapartum morbidity. To summarize, apart from reducing the risk of stillbirth, delivery of women with insulin-treated diabetes at 38 weeks may impart other benefits, such as reduction in infant size and a lower incidence of shoulder dystocia [59]. Amniocentesis to document fetal lung maturity is appropriate if gestational age is uncertain or for elective delivery before 38 weeks' gestation.

*Mild, diet-treated gestational diabetes*

The risk of stillbirth is not elevated in women with diet-treated gestational diabetes. Incentive for elective labor induction in women with gestational diabetes is related to estimates of fetal weight. There are several studies of labor induction among women with fetuses suspected to be overgrown regardless of diabetes status. Sanchez-Ramos and colleagues [60] described a meta-analysis of 11 studies and found that elective labor induction was associated with an increased risk of cesarean delivery without a decrease in the rate of shoulder dystocia. Another study reported that elective induction of labor increased the cesarean delivery rate, and did not prevent shoulder dystocia in situations where estimated fetal weight was greater than the 90th percentile [61]. Finally, a randomized trial of 273 women without diabetes did not show a reduction in the cesarean delivery or neonatal morbidity rates after ultrasound identification of a fetus estimated to weigh between 4000 and 4500 g [62]. Overall, the practice of elective labor induction in women without diabetes but suspected of fetal macrosomia yields no detectable benefits to the mother or fetus. However, the obstetric provider is often tempted to consider early elective delivery in women with gestational diabetes to avoid the increased risk of fetal overgrowth and difficult delivery. The evidence to justify such an intervention, however, is also lacking. In a review of randomized trials of elective delivery in women with diabetes from the Cochrane database, including those with mild gestational diabetes, there was little evidence to support elective labor induction [63]. Current available literature suggests that, while elective labor induction for women who have mild gestational diabetes may not result in a significant increase in maternal or fetal risk, the benefit of this practice remains unclear [64]. Amniocentesis to document fetal lung maturity for elective delivery before 39 weeks' gestation is recommended [65].

## When to perform a cesarean delivery

Cesarean delivery rates in women with either preexisting or gestational diabetes are uniformly increased [9,24]. For example, the cesarean delivery rate in women with overt diabetes has remained at about 80% for the past 25 years at Parkland Hospital [66]. Labor dystocia attributable to a large fetus is not the only factor that contributes to the high cesarean delivery rates in women with diabetes. Other factors include labor induction for maternal and fetal complications or the theoretical but unproven benefit of avoiding continued intrauterine growth and subsequent difficult delivery. As discussed previously, a policy of labor induction after 38 or 39 weeks of gestation in women with diet-treated gestational diabetes has not been proven beneficial but, other than the potential of an unnecessarily increased cesarean delivery rate, it is generally regarded as a safe practice.

Prophylactic primary cesarean delivery before labor using lower esti-mated fetal weight thresholds in women with diabetes has been proposed. Such a practice among women with diabetes is controversial and recommen-dations regarding estimated fetal weight thresholds for triggering primary cesarean delivery vary from 4000 to 4500 g. Specifically, some advocate ce-sarean delivery when the estimated fetal weight is at or exceeds 4000 g [67]. Others recommend 4250 g [68,69]. The American College of Obstetricians and Gynecologists establishes a threshold of 4500 g [70]. Complicating this practice are limitations in accurately estimating fetal weight [71,72]. The obvious consequence of this inaccuracy is an excess of unnecessary ce-sarean deliveries in women with diabetes, an increase in cesarean-associated maternal morbidity, and an overall increase in health care costs. For exam-ple, a study by Takoudes and colleagues [73] reported that women with pre-gestational diabetes, either Type 1 or 2, were 2.7 times more likely to have a wound infection when compared with the women without diabetes. Fur-ther, in a well-done cost analysis, an additional 153 cesarean deliveries in women with diabetes and an ultrasound-estimated fetal weight of 4500 g, (costing an extra $300,000) would need to be performed to prevent one per-manent brachial plexus injury [74]. Notably, although cesarean delivery can nearly eliminate the risk of shoulder dystocia [75], the risk of brachial plexus injury cannot be entirely eliminated. As shown in a recent large observa-tional study of cesarean deliveries, not all cases of brachial plexus injury fol-low a difficult vaginal delivery [76].

To summarize, for a woman whose pregnancy is complicated by diabetes and whose fetus is estimated to be at least 4500 g, a policy of primary cesar-ean section seems justified. A woman with diabetes whose fetus is estimated to be less than 4000 g should not be considered a candidate for cesarean de-livery based solely on fetal size. Importantly, in women with diabetes and a history of shoulder dystocia, primary cesarean delivery should be seriously considered. In women with diabetes and an estimated fetal weight between 4000 and 4500 g, routine elective cesarean delivery remains an area of con-troversy. Prior delivery history, clinical assessments of the maternal pelvis, and labor progress should be considered before proceeding with a cesarean delivery in these women.

## Intrapartum/peripartum glycemic management

Women with diabetes should not take long-acting insulin on the day of labor induction or elective cesarean delivery. Regular insulin may be used during labor as part of an infusion adjusted according to a capillary blood glucose monitoring–based protocol (Table 2). Capillary blood glucose values are checked hourly in certain action labor. The American College of Obstetrics and Gynecology suggests that hourly glucose levels be kept at less than 110 mg/dL [77]. In pregnancy, hyperglycemia promotes insulin secretion by the fetal pancreas. After delivery, when the newborn is no

Table 2
Protocol for insulin infusion during labor at Parkland Hospital

| CBG (mg per dL) | Insulin[a] (units per hour) | Fluids (rate = 125 mL per hour) |
|---|---|---|
| <100 | 0 | D5 Lactated Ringer Solution |
| 100 to 140 | 1 | D5 Lactated Ringer Solution |
| 141 to 180 | 1.5 | Normal saline |
| 181 to 220 | 2 | Normal saline |
| >220 | 2.5 | Normal saline |

*Abbreviation:* CBG, Capillary Blood Glucose, performed hourly.
[a] Dilute 25 units of regular insulin in 250 milliliters normal saline.

longer exposed to high maternal glycemic levels, neonatal hypoglycemia may result, with subsequent admission to the neonatal intensive care unit. Tight regulation of maternal glucose levels during labor can reduce the incidence of neonatal hypoglycemia, even among women with poor antepartum glycemic control [78]. The long-term implications of neonatal hypoglycemia on neurodevelopment remain unclear [79]. Women with diet-treated gestational diabetes generally do not require such intense monitoring and insulin therapy during labor.

## Summary

Diabetes in pregnancy confers a number of risks for both the mother and her baby, and many of these risks are encountered in the labor and delivery unit. The obstetric provider caring for women with diabetes should be alert to the risk of hypertension and the potential for difficult delivery as a result of the overgrown fetus. Women with preexisting diabetes or poor glycemic control are at increased risk for poor obstetrical outcomes such as stillbirth or delivery of a malformed infant.

To avoid difficult delivery of an overgrown infant, some have recommended early induction of labor or prophylactic cesarean delivery. Although controversial, there is some evidence that induction at 38 weeks in women with insulin-treated diabetes may reduce the rate of shoulder dystocia and delivery of large-for-gestational age neonates. On the other hand, prophylactic cesarean delivery has not been shown to improve perinatal outcomes. It is appropriate for the obstetric provider to consider the option of cesarean delivery in a woman whose pregnancy is complicated by diabetes and who is carrying a fetus with an estimated fetal weight of 4500 g or more. Meticulous attention to avoiding maternal hyperglycemia during labor can prevent neonatal hypoglycemia.

## References

[1] O'Sullivan JB. Gestational diabetes. Unsuspected, asymptomatic diabetes in pregnancy. N Engl J Med 1961;264:1082–5.

[2] Dandrow RV, O'Sullivan JB. Obstetric hazards of gestational diabetes. Am J Obstet Gynecol 1966;96:1144–7.

[3] O'Sullivan JB, Gellis SS, Dandrow RV, et al. The potential diabetic and her treatment in pregnancy. Obstet Gynecol 1966;27:683–9.

[4] Coustan DR, Lewis SB. Insulin therapy for gestational diabetes. Obstet Gynecol 1978;51: 306–10.

[5] Thompson DJ, Porter KB, Gunnells DJ, et al. Prophylactic insulin in the management of gestational diabetes. Obstet Gynecol 1990;75:960–4.

[6] Coustan DR, Imarah J. Prophylactic insulin treatment of gestational diabetes reduces the incidence of macrosomia, operative delivery and birth trauma. Am J Obstet Gynecol 1984;150:836–42.

[7] Langer O, Rodriguez DA, Xenakis EMJ, et al. Intensified versus conventional management of gestational diabetes. Am J Obstet Gynecol 1994;170:1036–47.

[8] Gabbe SG, Mestman H, Freeman RK, et al. Mangement and outcome of class A diabetes mellitus. Am J Obstet Gynecol 1977;127:465–9.

[9] Gabbe SG, Mestman JH, Freeman RK, et al. Management and outcome of pregnancy in diabetes mellitus, Classes B to R. Am J Obstet Gynecol 1977;129:723–32.

[10] Langer O, Levy J, Brustman L, et al. Glycemic control in gestational diabetes mellitus—how tight is tight enough: small for gestational age versus large for gestational age? Am J Obstet Gynecol 1989;161:646–53.

[11] Crowther CA, Hiller JE, Moss JR, et al. Effect treatment of gestational diabetes mellitus on pregnancy outcomes. N Engl J Med 2005;352:2477–86.

[12] Joffe GM, Esterlitz JR, Levine RJ, et al. The relationship between abnormal glucose tolerance and hypertensive disorders of pregnancy in healthy nulliparous women. Am J Obstet Gynecol 1998;179:1032–7.

[13] Yang X, Hsu-Hage B, Zhang H, et al. Women with impaired glucose tolerance during pregnancy have significantly poor pregnancy outcomes. Diabetes Care 2002;25: 1619–24.

[14] Stamilio DM, Olsen T, Ratcliffe S, et al. False-positive 1-hour glucose challenge test and adverse perinatal outcomes. Obstet Gynecol 2004;103:148–56.

[15] Yogev Y, Langer O, Xenakis EM, et al. The association between glucose challenge test, obesity and pregnancy outcome in 6390 non-diabetic women. J Matern Fetal Neonatal Med 2005;17:29–34.

[16] Lindsay MK, Graves W, Klein L. The relationship of one abnormal glucose tolerance test value and pregnancy complications. Obstet Gynecol 1989;73:103–6.

[17] Sermer M, Naylor CD, Gare DJ, et al. Impact of increasing carbohydrate intolerance on maternal-fetal outcomes in 3637 women without gestational diabetes. Am J Obstet Gynecol 1995;173:146–56.

[18] Jensen DM, Damm P, Sorensen B, et al. Clinical impact of mild carbohydrate intolerance in pregnancy: a study of 2904 nondiabetic Danish women with risk factors for gestational diabetes mellitus. Am J Obstet Gynecol 2001;185:413–9.

[19] McLaughlin GB, Cheng YW, Caughey AB. Women with one elevated 3-hour glucose tolerance test value: are they at risk for adverse perinatal outcomes? Am J Obstet Gynecol 2006; 194:e16–9.

[20] Gabbe SG, Graves CR. Management of diabetes complicating pregnancy. Obstet Gynecol 2003;102:857–68.

[21] Langer O, Conway DL. Level of glycemia and perinatal outcome in pregestational diabetes. J Matern Fetal Med 2000;9:35–41.

[22] Langer O, Yogev Y, Xenakis EM, et al. Overweight and obese in gestational diabetes: the impact on pregnancy outcome. Am J Obstet Gynecol 2005;192:1768–76.

[23] Garner P. Type I diabetes mellitus and pregnancy. Lancet 1995;346:157–61.

[24] Casey BM, Lucas MJ, McIntire DD, et al. Pregnancy outcomes in women with gestational diabetes compared with the general obstetric population. Obstet Gynecol 1997;90:869–73.

[25] Gregory KD, Henry OA, Ramicone E, et al. Maternal and infant complications in high and normal weight infants by method of delivery. Obstet Gynecol 1998;92:507–13.

[26] Lipscomb KR, Gregory K, Shaw K. The outcome of macrosomic infants weighing at least 4500 grams: Los Angeles County + University of Southern California experience. Obstet Gynecol 1995;85:558–64.

[27] Nesbitt TS, Gilbert WM, Herrchen B. Shoulder dystocia and associated risk factors with macrosomic infants born in California. Am J Obstet Gynecol 1998;179:476–80.

[28] Naylor CD, Sermer M, Chen E, et al. Cesarean delivery in relation to birth weight and gestational glucose tolerance: pathophysiology or practice style? JAMA 1996;275:1165–70.

[29] Mazouni C, Porcu G, Cohen-Solal E, et al. Maternal and anthropomorphic risk factors for shoulder dystocia. Acta Obstetrica et Gynecologica Scandinavica 2006;85:567–70.

[30] Ouzounian JG, Gherman RB. Shoulder dystocia: are historic risk factors reliable predictors? Am J Obstet Gynecol 2005;192:1933–8.

[31] Ray JG, Vermeulen MJ, Shapiro JL, et al. Maternal and neonatal outcomes in pregestational and gestational diabetes mellitus, and the influence of maternal obesity and weight gain: the DEPOSIT study. Diabetes Endocrine Pregnancy Outcome Study in Toronto. QJM 2001;94: 347–56.

[32] Greene JR, Soohoo SL. Factors associated with rectal injury in spontaneous deliveries. Obstet Gynecol 1989;73:732–8.

[33] Handa VL, Danielsen BH, Gilbert WM. Obstetric anal sphincter lacerations. Obstet Gynecol 2001;98:225–30.

[34] Fenner DE, Genberg B, Brahma P, et al. Fecal and urinary incontinence after vaginal delivery with anal sphincter disruption in an obstetrics unit in the United States. Am J Obstet Gynecol 2003;189:1543–9.

[35] Casey BM, Schaffer JI, Bloom SL, et al. Obstetric antecedents for postpartum pelvic floor dysfunction. Am J Obstet Gynecol 2005;192:1655–62.

[36] Buchsbaum GM, Duecy EE, Kerr LA, et al. Urinary incontinence in nulliparous women and their parous sisters. Obstet Gynecol 2005;106:1253–8.

[37] Persson J, Wolner-Hanssen P, Rydhstroem H. Obstetric risk factors for stress urinary incontinence. A population-based study. Obstet Gynecol 2000;96:440–5.

[38] Sibai BM, Caritis S, Hauth J. Risks of preeclampsia and adverse neonatal outcomes among women with pregestational diabetes mellitus. Am J of Obstet Gynecol 2000;182:364–9.

[39] Innes KE, Wimsatt JH, McDuffie R. Relative glucose tolerance and subsequent development of hypertension in pregnancy. Obstet Gynecol 2001;97:905–10.

[40] Bartha JL, Martinez-Del-Fresno P, Comino-Delgado R. Gestational diabetes mellitus diagnosed during early pregnancy. Am J Obstet Gynecol 2000;182:346–50.

[41] Yogev Y, Xenakis EM, Langer O. The association between preeclampsia and the severity of gestational diabetes: the impact of glycemic control. Am J Obstet Gynecol 2004;191: 1655–60.

[42] Macintosh MC, Fleming KM, Bailey JA, et al. Perinatal mortality and congenital anomalies in babies of women with type 1 or type 2 diabetes in England, Wales, and Northern Ireland: population-based study. BMJ 2006;333:177.

[43] Pearson DW, Kernaghan D, Lee R, et al. The relationship between pre-pregnancy care and early pregnancy loss, major congenital anomaly or perinatal death in type I diabetes mellitus. BJOG 2007;114:104–7.

[44] Jensen DM, Damm P, Moelsted-Pedersen L, et al. Outcomes in type 1 diabetic pregnancies: a nationwide, population-based study. Diabetes Care 2004;27:2819–23.

[45] Fretts RC, Boyd ME, Usher RH, et al. The changing pattern of fetal death, 1961–1988. Obstet Gynecol 1992;79:35–9.

[46] Lauenborg J, Mathiesen E, Ovesen P, et al. Audit on stillbirths in women with pregestational type 1 diabetes. Diabetes Care 2003;26:1385–9.

[47] Galindo A, Burguillo AG, Azriel S, et al. Outcome of fetuses with pregestational diabetes mellitus. J Perinat Med 2006;34:323–31.

[48] Li R, Chase M, Jung SK, et al. Hypoxic stress in diabetic pregnancy contributes to impaired embryo gene expression and defective development by inducing oxidative stress. Am J Physiol Endocrinol Metab 2005;289(4):E591–9.
[49] Loeken MR. Advances in understanding the molecular causes of diabetes-induced birth defects. J Soc Gynecol Investig 2006;13(1):2–10.
[50] Sheffield JS, Butler-Koster EL, Casey BM, et al. Maternal diabetes mellitus and infant malformations. Obstet Gynecol 2002;100:925–30.
[51] Miller E, Hare JW, Cloherty JP, et al. Elevated maternal hemoglobin A1c in early pregnancy and major congenital anomalies in infants of diabetic mothers. N Engl J Med 1981;304:1331–4.
[52] Greene MF, Hare JW, Cloherty JP, et al. First-trimester hemoglobin A1 and risk for major malformation and spontaneous abortion in diabetic pregnancy. Teratology 1989;39:225–31.
[53] Lucas MJ, Leveno KJ, Williams ML, et al. Early pregnancy glycosylated hemoglobin, severity of diabetes, and fetal malformations. Am J Obstet Gynecol 1989;161:426–31.
[54] Klinke JA, Toth EL. Preconception care for women with type I diabetes. Can Fam Physician 2003;49:769–73.
[55] American College of Obstetricians and Gynecologists. Neural tube defects. Practice Bulletin Number 44. 2003.
[56] Anteby EY, Yagel S. Route of delivery of fetuses with structural anomalies. Eur J Obstet Gynecol Reprod Biol 2003;106:5–9.
[57] Kjos SL, Henry OA, Montoro M, et al. Insulin-requiring diabetes in pregnancy: a randomized trial of active induction of labor and expectant management. Am J Obstet Gynecol 1993;169:611–5.
[58] Rayburn WF, Sokkary N, Clokey DE, et al. Consequences of routine delivery at 38 weeks for A-2 gestational diabetes. J Matern Fetal Neonatal Med 2005;18:333–7.
[59] Lurie S, Insler V, Hagay ZJ. Induction of labor at 38 to 39 weeks of gestation reduces the incidence of shoulder dystocia in gestational diabetic patients Class A2. Am J Perinatol 1996;13:293–6.
[60] Sanchez-Ramos L, Bernstein S, Kaunitz AM. Expectant management versus labor induction for suspected fetal macrosomia: a systematic review. Obstet Gynecol 2002;100:997–1002.
[61] Combs CA, Singh NB, Khoury JC. Elective induction versus spontaneous labor after sonographic diagnosis of fetal macrosomia. Obstet Gynecol 1993;81:492–6.
[62] Gonen O, Rosen DJD, Dolfin Z, et al. Induction of labor versus expectant management in macrosomia: a randomized study. Obstet Gynecol 1997;89:913–7.
[63] Boulvain M, Stan C, Irion O. Elective delivery in diabetic pregnant women. Cochrane Database Syst Rev 2001;2:CD001997.
[64] Sacks DA, Sacks A. Induction of labor versus conservative management of pregnant diabetic women. J Matern Fetal Neonatal Med 2002;12:438–41.
[65] American College of Obstetrics and Gynecology. Assessment of fetal lung maturity. Educational Bulletin Number 230. 1996.
[66] Cunningham FG, Leveno KJ, Bloom SL, et al. Williams Obstetrics. 22nd edition. New York: McGraw-Hill; 2005.
[67] Acker DB, Sachs BP, Friedman EA. Risk factors for shoulder dystocia. Obstet Gynecol 1985;66:762–8.
[68] Langer O, Berkus MD, Huff RW, et al. Shoulder dystocia: should the fetus weighing greater than or equal to 4000 grams be delivered by cesarean section? Am J Obstet Gynecol 1991;165:831–7.
[69] Conway DL, Langer O. Elective delivery of infants with macrosomia in diabetic women: reduced shoulder dystocia versus increased cesarean deliveries. Am J Obstet Gynecol 1998;178:922–5.
[70] American College of Obstetrics and Gynecology. Shoulder dystocia. practice Bulletin Number 40. 2002.

334    HAWKINS & CASEY

[71] Gonen R, Spiegel D, Abend M. Is macrosomia predictable, and are shoulder dystocia and birth trauma preventable? Obstet Gynecol 1996;88:526–9.
[72] Landon MB. Prenatal diagnosis of macrosomia in pregnancy complicated by diabetes mellitus. J Matern Fetal Med 2000;9:52–4.
[73] Takoudes TC, Weitzen S, Slocum J, et al. Risk of cesarean wound complications in diabetic gestations. Am J Obstet Gynecol 2004;191:958–63.
[74] Rouse DJ, Owen J, Goldenberg RL, et al. The effectiveness and costs of elective cesarean delivery for fetal macrosomia diagnosed by ultrasound. JAMA 1996;276:1480–6.
[75] Conway DL. Delivery of the macrosomic infant: cesarean section versus vaginal delivery. Semin Perinatol 2002;26:225–31.
[76] Alexander JM, Leveno KJ, Hauth J, et al. Fetal injury associated with cesarean delivery. Obstet Gynecol 2006;108:885–90.
[77] American College of Obstetrics and Gynecology. Pregestational diabetes mellitus. Practice Bulletin Number 60. 2005.
[78] Curet LB, Izquierdo LA, Gilson GJ, et al. Relative effects of antepartum and intrapartum maternal blood glucose levels on incidence of neonatal hypoglycemia. J Perinatol 1997;17(2):113–5.
[79] Boluyt N, van Kempen A, Offringa M. Neurodevelopment after neonatal hypoglycemia: a systematic review and design of an optimal future study. Pediatrics 2006;117(6):2231–43.

ELSEVIER
SAUNDERS

Obstet Gynecol Clin N Am
34 (2007) 335–349

OBSTETRICS AND
GYNECOLOGY
CLINICS
OF NORTH AMERICA

# After Pregnancy Complicated by Diabetes: Postpartum Care and Education

## Siri L. Kjos, MD

*Department of Obstetrics and Gynecology, Harbor UCLA Medical Center,*
*1000 West Carson Street, Box 3A, Torrance, CA 90509, USA*

During the puerperium, the physician has a unique opportunity to encourage new mothers with either pregestational or gestational diabetes (GDM) to make permanent the positive changes in lifestyle, diet, and medical therapy they adopted during pregnancy. Success in making such a transition into the interconception period may ultimately have far-reaching effects on her quality of life, her offspring's risk for diabetes, and her subsequent pregnancy outcome. To be most successful in preparing for this transition, education should begin during pregnancy and should address three care issues:

How she can best reduce the risk of obesity, metabolic syndrome, and diabetes in her newborn by breastfeeding and instituting healthy lifestyle goals for her child
How she can best minimize her risk for developing diabetes or complications of diabetes through lifestyle changes and medical care to control hyperglycemia
How she can control her reproductive health through effective contraception and planning of subsequent pregnancies

During hospitalization after delivery, the mother and her physician can begin to develop and institute care plans for her baby and herself.

## The immediate puerperium

*Management of glucose during hospitalization*

With the delivery of the placenta, the marked insulin resistance of pregnancy abruptly disappears, resulting in a variable period of improved insulin

---

*E-mail address:* skjos@obgyn.humc.edu

0889-8545/07/$ - see front matter © 2007 Elsevier Inc. All rights reserved.
doi:10.1016/j.ogc.2007.04.004
*obgyn.theclinics.com*

sensitivity for women with all types of diabetes. Women with type 1 diabetes often require very little insulin during the first 24 to 72 hours following delivery. During this period, especially following operative delivery, their insulin needs are variable, and insulin dosing is best accomplished using a premeal sliding scale. Afterwards, when regular eating patterns resume, women with multiple dose therapy or continuous insulin infusion generally require a one-third to one-half reduction from pregnancy insulin doses (ie, the insulin/carbohydrate ratio used for premeal short-acting insulin dose/bolus and the long-acting insulin/basal infusion rates need to be reduced). Type 1 women on fixed split doses can generally be restarted at about 0.6 total daily units of insulin per kilogram of postpartum weight, giving two thirds of the total dose prebreakfast (one third short-acting and two thirds intermediate-acting [NPH]) and one third of total dose in the evening. The evening dose of short and intermediate acting can be given together or further split to a predinner dose of short-acting (one half of evening dose) and a before-bedtime dose of intermediate-acting NPH (one half of evening dose). Postpartum glycemic targets can be relaxed to fasting and postprandial targets of 100 and 150 mg/dL, respectively. Women with type 2 diabetes often have adequate glycemic control immediately following delivery and may not require any medical therapy during hospitalization. These women can be followed with daily fasting capillary glucose levels during hospitalization and after discharge. If resumption of oral antihyperglycemic agents is necessary, glyburide, glipizide [1], or metformin [2–4] have been shown to have little or no transfer into human milk and can be prescribed for breastfeeding women, with counseling.

In most cases, glycemic control in women with GDM normalizes and glucose monitoring in the hospital can cease after the establishment of a normal fasting glucose level ($<100$ mg/dL) [5]. Women with GDM can have a wide spectrum of glucose intolerance, ranging from transient, mild intolerance, which may be limited to pregnancy, to probable, unrecognized diabetes, which may have antedated pregnancy. Risk factors for persistent diabetes include pregnancy fasting glucose levels greater than or equal to 126 mg/dL (ie, meeting nonpregnant criteria for diagnosis of diabetes); diagnosis of GDM during the first trimester; and a prior history of GDM without documented normal glucose tolerance outside of pregnancy [6]. A small subset of women with GDM will have overt hyperglycemia after delivery and can be diagnosed by the presence of fasting hyperglycemia. The diagnosis of diabetes requires at least two overnight fasting serum glucose levels greater than or equal to 126 mg/dL in an ambulatory setting, and should not be made while the patient is postoperative or recovering from an infection [5]. Insulin therapy is generally not indicated unless marked fasting hyperglycemia (200–250 mg/dL) is present. Women with less elevated fasting glucose levels (100–199 mg/dL) can be discharged home, and fasting glucose levels monitored with early follow-up 1 to 2 weeks after delivery to establish the diagnosis of diabetes and institute medical therapy as needed.

In women with type 1 diabetes, a daily schedule for pre- or postprandial glucose monitoring should be established before discharge. Working with her internist, a plan for euglycemic management should be developed. Guidelines for the frequency of self-monitoring of blood glucose (SMBG) for type 2 diabetes are less well established [5] and depend on the patient's glucose control, medical therapy, and motivation, and the recommendations of her internist. Daily or twice-weekly fasting capillary glucose levels during the 6 to 8 weeks after delivery will provide valuable information about the need to start or adjust medical therapy and for assessing compliance with diet recommendations. For women who were not receiving regular care for their diabetes before pregnancy, a referral for continued diabetic care should be made.

*Dietary counseling*

During hospitalization, a medical nutritional consult should be obtained for all women with pre-existing or GDM. Her total daily caloric needs should be recalculated, based on her healthy weight target and breastfeeding needs. General guidelines for postpartum caloric intake are about 25 kcal/kg/d and 27 to 30 kcal/kg/d in nonbreastfeeding and breastfeeding women, respectively [7].

*Breastfeeding*

The American Academy of Pediatrics [8] and the Surgeon General [9] strongly recommend exclusive breastfeeding for at least the first 6 months of life, and preferably for the first 12 months. GDM or pregestational diabetes is not a contraindication to breastfeeding. Prenatal education is important and the mother should follow peripartum hospital policies and practices, which encourage early breastfeeding after delivery and minimization of the separation of mother and infant postdelivery. Early postpartum follow-up 1 to 2 weeks after delivery is helpful in assessing changing glycemic control in type 1 and 2 diabetic women, so that medical therapy may be instituted if needed. Early visits also allow the physician to identify problems with breastfeeding and to encourage the following of dietary and exercise guidelines.

## Reduction of later childhood obesity and carbohydrate intolerance risk for the newborn infant

*Education*

Increasingly, evidence has accumulated that the offspring of diabetic mothers are at increased risk for childhood obesity and for type 2 diabetes later in life. Several studies [10] that included various ethnic groups such as native Americans [11] and European Caucasian women with GDM [12] suggest that breastfed infants are at a lower risk of later developing obesity or diabetes. A longer duration of exclusive breastfeeding and a later introduction of formula may also be protective of developing β-cell autoimmunity, and later risk for type 1 diabetes [13]. Although long-term, prospective studies in this population are lacking, sufficient data suggest that the benefits of breastfeeding may be of greater importance to infants of diabetic mothers than the general health benefits of breastfeeding to the newborn. Due to the higher likelihood of operative delivery and immediate separation from their neonate after birth with diabetic pregnancies, there may be initial difficulties with breastfeeding [14]. Encouragement and assistance with lactation instruction can overcome most problems. In diabetic women who have good metabolic control, the quality of breast milk is not substantially affected [15,16]. One study found lower fasting glucose levels and adequate caloric intake (31 kcal/kg) to be associated with successful continuation of lactation beyond 6 weeks in women with type 1 diabetes [17]. In women with prior GDM who continued to breastfeed, lower fasting glucose levels and lower rates of diabetes were also found, compared with nonbreastfeeding women, 1 to 3 months after delivery [18].

Equally important is maternal education to prevent childhood obesity, a forerunner of type 2 diabetes in young adults. The dietary and lifestyle guidelines the mothers are encouraged to follow should be extended to their offspring. National [19] and state childhood obesity prevention programs exist to help families and health care providers. The new mother should be encouraged to inform her child's pediatrician about her diabetes status and discuss preventive lifestyle measures she can institute for her child. The American Diabetes Association has guidelines for screening high-risk children and adolescents for future type 2 diabetes [20].

## Reduction of risk for developing diabetes or complications of diabetes

*Education and medical care for women with type 1 and 2 diabetes*

After completing a pregnancy with strict glycemic control, diabetic mothers have the tools and experience needed to optimize glucose control. They should be encouraged to continue their positive health habits from pregnancy. The "ABCs" of diabetes should be stressed: $A_{1c}$ (controlling glucose [hemoglobin $A_{1c}$]), Blood pressure, and Cholesterol. They should be encouraged to make a commitment to maintain normal glucose levels; it should be explained that this will prevent, or slow progression of, diabetic sequelae. Large, controlled, prospective clinical trials in both type 1 [21] and type 2 [22] diabetes have demonstrated that strict glycemic control significantly cuts in half the risk for microvascular complications (ie, retinopathy, nephropathy, and neuropathy). The risk reduction is continuous without a discernable threshold. In type 1 diabetics, intensive therapy reduced the development and progression of retinopathy by 76% and 54%, respectively, microalbuminuria and nephropathy by 39% and 54%, respectively, and clinical neuropathy by 60% [17]. The intensive therapy followed was similar to that recommended during pregnancy, using continuous insulin infusion or three to four daily injections of insulin and frequent SMBG. Similarly, studies in nonpregnant patients who had type 2 diabetes, in which intensive medical therapy normalized glucose levels using mono- or a combo-therapy of insulin, sulfonylureas, or metformin, found a 25% reduction in microvascular complications [10]. Similar to type 1 diabetes, the relationship between glycemia and rate of complications in type 2 diabetes was also continuous: each percentage point drop in glycosylated hemoglobin levels was associated with a reduction in microvascular complications (35%), diabetes-related deaths (25%), and myocardial infarctions (18%) [23–25].

To achieve this degree of risk reduction, patients who have type 1 diabetes require frequent SMBG at least three to four times a day, with at least three daily injections of insulin [5]. The optimal frequency of glycemic monitoring of type 2 diabetic patients has not been established, but it should be sufficient to achieve glycemic control. Glycemic goals for both types of diabetes are similar (ie, preprandial glucose levels of 80 to 120 mg/dL and before-bed levels of 100 to 140 mg/dL and $HbA_{1c}$ below 7% [5]). Glycemic management in type 2 diabetes should be monitored every 3 months with $HbA_{1c}$ levels, adding SMBG in a stepwise fashion as glucose levels and more intensive therapy is required [12,13]. Preprandial and bedtime glucose levels above 140 and 160 mg/dL or $HbA_{1c}$ above 8% should trigger more intensive management, a change in therapy, or referral for further diabetic care [5]. At every visit, the role of the obstetrician-gynecologist should be to review his/her patient's compliance with her diabetic therapy and her level of glycemic control, reiterating the importance of euglycemia in reducing the risk of diabetic sequelae for her and the risk of congenital malformations in her future offspring [26].

Control of blood pressure (systolic less than or equal to 130 mmHg, diastolic less than 80 mmHg) is equally important to prevent cardiovascular and microvascular complications. Again, this control is accomplished by diet and exercise to achieve a healthy weight, adding medical therapy as needed [27]. Angiotensin-converting enzyme inhibitor or angiotensin receptor blockers are the preferred medication in diabetic patients because their use has been shown to delay the progression of nephropathy [5]. These agents have recently been shown to be teratogenic and should be discontinued before pregnancy; the patient should switch to another agent during the preconception period [28].

Normalizing serum lipid levels prevents macrovascular disease. Evaluation of fasting lipid profiles is best delayed 3 to 6 months after delivery to avoid the physiologic elevated low-density lipoprotein cholesterol levels associated with pregnancy [29]. They should be assessed at least annually in diabetic women. The primary treatment again is diet and exercise, adding medical therapy as needed [30].

*Education and medical care in women with prior gestational diabetes*

Women with GDM have a 50% to 60% lifetime risk for developing diabetes, mostly commonly type 2. Many identifiable clinical factors have been associated with developing diabetes within 5 years after pregnancy, including most measures of serum glucose during, or after, pregnancy (eg, the fasting, 1-hour, 2-hour glucose level; area under the glucose curve of the pregnancy; or postpartum oral glucose tolerance test [OGTT]); poor β-cell function; obesity (eg, prepregnancy or postpartum body mass index and weight gain during or after pregnancy); and indicators for a longer period of glucose intolerance (eg, earlier gestational age at diagnosis and previous GDM). In a review by Kim and colleagues [31] of studies in which follow-up OGTTs were performed after delivery in women with GDM using National Diabetes Data Group criteria, an elevated fasting pregnancy glucose level was the most commonly reported risk factor for developing diabetes. One study found a 21-fold risk of postpartum diabetes (36.7%) when any fasting pregnancy plasma glucose exceeded 121 mg/dL, compared with fasting levels remaining below 95 mg/dL [32]. When β-cell function is measured concurrently [33], fasting glucose levels decrease in predictive ability, which suggests that once fasting glucose levels during pregnancy become elevated, the rates of declining β-cell reserve and developing diabetes progress at a similar linear rate. In the review by Kim and colleagues [31], when studies were adjusted for dropouts and length of follow-up, the initial variable rates among different ethnic groups for the progression of diabetes were nearly eliminated. Postpartum impaired glucose tolerance (IGT) has also been found to an excellent independent predictor of subsequent diabetes in different ethnic groups [34,35] and identifies a high-risk group for preventive lifestyle and medical therapy. Postpartum impaired fasting glucose and impaired glucose tolerance appear to have a poor concordance [36]. Impaired fasting glucose levels may identify patients with different risk profiles, having a stronger association with metabolic syndrome, higher body mass index, central obesity, hypertension, and abnormal lipids [37].

The recent Fifth International Workshop Conference on GDM recommended that the postpartum glycemic status of women with recent GDM should be established 6 weeks postpartum using a 75-g, 2-hour OGTT, repeated in 1 year and then at minimum every 3 years thereafter [38]. The use of OGTT was endorsed by the Conference because of the low sensitivity of fasting plasma glucose (FPG) alone to detect impaired glucose tolerance and diabetes. The diagnosis of diabetes is made either by FPG greater than or equal to 126 mg/dL delivery or by a 2-hour plasma glucose level greater than or equal to 200 mg/dL, both of which must be confirmed by a subsequent FPG greater than or equal to 126 mg/dL [5]. Women who develop impaired fasting glucose levels ($\geq 110$ and $< 126$ mg/dL) or impaired glucose tolerance (IGT; 2-hour plasma glucose $\geq 140$ and $< 200$ mg/dL) are at greatest risk for developing subsequent diabetes [35,39]. Women with prior GDM and postpartum IGT have been shown to have a 16% annual incidence rate of developing diabetes [35].

During the last decade, randomized intervention trials have demonstrated that type 2 diabetes can be delayed or prevented in subjects with impaired glucose tolerance. Two controlled trials found intensive lifestyle interventions over 4 to 6 years reduced the diabetes risk by 58%, compared with nonintervention [40,41]. The antihyperglycemic agents metformin [40], acarbose [42], and orlistat [43] (the latter in addition to intensive lifestyle) have also been shown, although less successfully, to reduce the risk by 31%, 25%, and 37%, respectively. One randomized controlled trial conducted in high-risk Hispanic women with prior GDM found troglitazone to reduce the diabetes risk by 55% [44] and found that the protective mechanism was related to those who responded to the decrease in insulin resistance by reducing insulin secretion ("β-cell rest"). Although it is premature to recommend medical therapy for primary prevention of type 2 diabetes in women with prior GDM, ample support recommends active lifestyle changes, including structured exercise, healthy dietary changes, and weight loss programs.

*Lifestyle intervention*

Medical nutritional therapy to normalize blood glucose levels and provide adequate calories for maintaining or achieving normal or reasonable body weight is integral to diabetic care [45]. Similarly, the promotion of a daily exercise program, adjusted to the health status of the individual diabetic patient, is another vital component of diabetic care [46]. Recently, several clinical trials have demonstrated dietary and aerobic exercise programs to increase glucose use [47,48], improve lipid levels [49], decrease coagulation factors [50], and promote weight reduction [51] in patients who have type 2 diabetes. No studies have addressed dietary and exercise interventions to prevent diabetes in women with prior GDM. However, in a 12-year, primary prevention trial in Sweden, of 6956 middle-aged men undergoing glucose tolerance testing, those with IGT were randomized to either an intervention program of dietary counseling and physical exercise or to a routine treatment IGT group [51]. After 12 years, the mortality in the IGT intervention group was similar to that of subjects with normal glucose tolerance (6.5 versus 6.2 per 1000 person-years at risk) and significantly lower than the IGT routine treatment group (1.5 versus 14.0, $P = .009$) [51]. Furthermore, in subjects with IGT, the only significant predictor of mortality was the diet and exercise intervention. Body mass index, blood pressure, smoking, cholesterol, or the 2-hour glucose levels were not predictive. Similarly, a randomized, controlled, 6-year trial of 577 Chinese subjects with IGT found programs of active intervention with diet, exercise, and diet-plus-exercise were successful in reducing the adjusted risk of developing type 2 diabetes by 31%, 46%, and 42%, respectively [52]. These findings provide support for long-term lifestyle intervention programs in patients at high risk for type 2 diabetes (eg, those with IGT and, by extension, women with prior GDM). Economic models of prevention programs in women with prior GDM suggest such programs would save substantial health care dollars, because these women are already identified by their pregnancy as being at risk [53].

The postpartum period is an ideal time to initiate lifestyle changes because women are generally motivated to lose their pregnancy weight and are "fresh" from a regimen of intensive glycemic management. By continuing the American Diabetes Association diet, with appropriate caloric adjustments for achieving ideal body weight and additional calories required for lactation, little dietary re-education is required in women with GDM. Patients should be encouraged to implement similar dietary changes for their entire family, because their offspring are also at significantly increased risk for obesity and deteriorating glucose tolerance [54–60]. Exercise programs should encourage aerobic exercise, with the intensity of exercise adjusted to the patient's age, physical fitness, and health status, determined by a pre-exercise health evaluation [46]. Keeping in mind that many women with prior GDM are obese and sedentary, and that a program of minimal physical activity improves health [59,60], it may be more successful to begin with a simple exercise program, such as daily brisk walking for 10 to 15 minutes each day. This program should be increased to a minimum of 30 minutes per day of moderate physical activity as the patient gains conditioning [61]. Patients with better conditioning should be encouraged to engage in a program of more vigorous aerobic exercise.

## Reproductive health and contraception during the postpartum period

### Breastfeeding and contraception

With the delivery of the placenta, estrogen and progesterone levels immediately drop, removing the inhibitory effect of prolactin, and permitting breast milk production to begin. Three to four days after delivery, breast engorgement and full milk secretion starts. Newborn suckling further stimulates and maintains the release of prolactin, to sustain milk production. Prolactin also interrupts the cyclic release of gonadotropin-releasing hormone, which blocks the pulsatile release of luteinizing hormone, and thereby blocks follicle-stimulating, hormone-mediated stimulation of the ovary, and ovulation. The return of ovulation is delayed in breastfeeding women and the earliest return of ovulation has been documented to be 25 days after delivery in nonbreastfeeding women [62]. In nonbreastfeeding women, fertility can return by 4 weeks after delivery and contraception is advised. In exclusively breastfeeding women, ovulation is reliably delayed for up to 6 months, providing 98% efficacy in pregnancy protection [63–66]. Thus, all contraceptive methods used for the first 6 months in conjunction with exclusive breastfeeding have a low failure rate.

When exclusive breastfeeding is used as a birth control method, it is called the lactation amenorrhea method (LAM). When using LAM, women should begin breastfeeding immediately after delivery and avoid supplementation, and they need to breastfeed frequently (ie, at least every 4 hours during the daytime and 6 hours during nighttime). Another contraceptive method should be initiated if menses return, 6 months have elapsed since delivery, or supplementing feeding is used. The 6-month cumulative pregnancy rate using LAM is up to 1.2% (95% CI, 0%–2.4%) [67].

Contraceptive needs should be discussed during the postpartum visit. Frequency of intercourse is often diminished from the demands of motherhood. Women may be reluctant to take any medication while breastfeeding for fear of exposing their newborn to medication. For women with diabetes or recent GDM, a strong endorsement of breastfeeding can be coupled with LAM plus condoms. This combination will effectively provide pregnancy protection and encourage exclusive breastfeeding, which, among the health benefits for their newborn, may also reduce childhood obesity and glucose intolerance risk.

For women who desire hormonal contraception, they can be reassured that the level of hormone transferred to breast milk, less than 1% of maternal dose, is comparable to hormone levels observed during ovulatory cycles. Progestin-only methods generally are favored because they have no demonstrable effect on milk volume, whereas the effect of a combination of estrogen and progestin oral contraceptives (OCs) is inconclusive [67]. No effect has been found on infant growth and weight with either progestin-only methods or combined oral contraceptive (COC) use. Expert committees [68–70] recommend that when women are breastfeeding and desire hormonal contraception, progestin-only OCs can be started on day 21 postpartum with additional protection if needed, and COCs should not be started before 6 weeks postpartum, after thromboembolic risk is normalized, lactation is well established, and the infant's nutritional status is well monitored [70]. The World Health Organization [68] discourages COC use until after 6 months to encourage breastfeeding. Progestin-only injectable methods (eg, depo-medroxyprogesterone acetate) are not recommended until 6 weeks postdelivery [70] but may be given as early as 21 days postpartum if the risk of immediate pregnancy is high [69]. Emergency contraception, given within 72 hours of unprotected coitus, is not indicated before 21 days postpartum, after which time the standard use guidelines can be followed.

*Hormonal contraception and diabetes*

Planning a subsequent pregnancy while in optimal glycemic control and health is essential for women with type 1 and 2 diabetes and requires effective contraception. Only then can they reduce their future offspring's risk of congenital malformations [71,72]. Planned pregnancy, after the assessment of glycemic status in women with prior GDM, is also important. Unrecognized and untreated hyperglycemia (FPG > 120 mg/dL) detected during pregnancy has been shown to more than double the risk for major congenital malformations [73].

The short-term use of low-dose COCs [74–77] and progestin-only OCs [74] in women with type 1 diabetes appears to produce minimal metabolic effects. Long-term prospective studies evaluating the effect of OC use on

KJOS

diabetic sequelae are lacking. However, retrospective, cross-sectional studies [78] and case-control trials [79] in women with type 1 diabetes have not found any increased risk of, or progression of, retinopathy, renal disease, or hypertension with past or current use of OCs.

In women with prior GDM, short-term studies have shown a minimal effect of low-dose COCs on carbohydrate and lipid metabolism [80–82]. Longer-term use does not appear to increase the risk of developing diabetes. A large controlled trial found virtually identical 3-year diabetes cumulative incidence rates with uninterrupted use of low-dose COCs (25.4%) and nonhormonal contraception (26.5%) [83]. In contrast, the use of the progestin-only OCs while breastfeeding increased diabetic risk almost threefold and this risk increased with longer duration of uninterrupted use [84]. In a recent study, the risk of diabetes was doubled in breastfeeding women with prior GDM using the long-acting injectable progestin, depo-medroxyprogesterone acetone, compared with nonbreastfeeding users of injectable progestin and COCs [84]. Thus, progestin-only methods should not be prescribed to women with prior GDM while they are breastfeeding. Alternatives include using LAM plus condoms or nonhormonal methods, or starting low-dose COCs 6 to 8 weeks postpartum. The lowest dose and potency progestin (and estrogen) combination OC should be selected to minimize adverse deterioration in glucose tolerance, lipid metabolism, and blood pressure effects in women with diabetes and prior GDM [85].

*Intrauterine device*

Intrauterine devices (IUDs) provide excellent long-acting pregnancy protection in diabetic women. Medicated copper IUDs have not been associated with any increase risk of pelvic inflammatory disease after the postinsertion period in healthy women [86] or in women with type 1 [87,88] or type 2 [89] diabetes. Data regarding diabetic women with progestin-medicated IUDs are not available. No contraindications exist to IUD use in women with prior GDM.

The copper medicated device can be inserted within 48 hours of delivery. Otherwise, insertion of copper-medicated IUDs and the levonorgestrel intrauterine system should be delayed to at least 4 weeks postpartum after involution of the uterus. Guidelines for the selection of proper candidates and for monitoring of IUD use in women with diabetes or prior GDM are similar to those for the general population. No studies in diabetic women used general prophylaxis with insertion or removal, and therefore it appears unlikely to add any benefit.

**Summary**

The postpartum period in women with pregestational or GDM allows the physician and mother to relax from the intensive medical and obstetric management and switch into a proactive and preventive mode, and jointly develop a reproductive health plan. The woman's individual needs regarding contraception and breastfeeding, an appropriate diet to achieve healthy weight goals, the medical management of diabetes, daily exercise, and future pregnancy planning must be considered. Essential is the active participation of the woman, who, through education, gains an understanding of the far-reaching effects her active participation will have on her subsequent health, her newborn child's health, and possibly that of her future children.

## References

[1] Feig DS, Briggs GG, Kraemer JM, et al. Transfer of glyburide and glipizide into breast milk. Diabetes Care 2005;28:1851–5.
[2] Hale TW, Kristensin JH, Hackett LP, et al. Transfer of metformin into human milk. Diabetologia 2004;45:1509–14.
[3] Gardiner SJ, Kirpatrick CMJ, Begg EJ, et al. Transfer of metformin into human milk. Clin Pharmocol Ther 2003;73:71077.
[4] Simmons D, Walters BNJ, Rowan JA, et al. Metformin therapy and diabetes in pregnancy. Med J Aust 2004;180:462–4.
[5] American Diabetes Association. Standards for medical care in diabetes—2007. Diabetes Care 2007;30(Suppl 1):S4–41.
[6] Metzger BE. Summary and recommendations of the 4th International Workshop-Conference on Gestational Diabetes Mellitus. Diabetes Care 1998;21(Suppl 2):B161–7.
[7] Jovanovic L, Nakai Y. Successful pregnancy in women with type 1 diabetes: from preconception through postpartum care. Endocrinol Metab Clin North Am 2006;35:79–97.
[8] American Academy Pediatrics Policy Statement. Breastfeeding the use of human milk. Pediatrics 2005;115:496–506.
[9] US Department of Health and Human Services. HSS blueprint for action on breastfeeding. Washington, DC: USDHHS, Office of Women's Health; 2000.
[10] Scialli AR. Public Affairs Committee of the Teratology Society. Teratology public affairs committee position paper: maternal obesity and pregnancy. Birth Defects Res A Clin Mol Teratol 2006;76:73–7.
[11] Young TK, Martens PJ, Taback SP, et al. Type 2 diabetes mellitus in children: prenatal and early infancy risk factors among native Canadians. Arch Pediatr Adolesc Med 2002;156:651–5.
[12] Schaefer-Graf U, Hartmann R, Pawliczak J, et al. Association of breast-feeding and early childhood overweight in children from mothers with gestational diabetes mellitus. Diabetes Care 2006;29:1105–7.
[13] Holmberg H, Wahlberg J, Vaarala O, et al, ABIS Study Group. Short duration of breast-feeding as a risk-factor for β-cell autoantiboides in 5-year-old children from the general population. Br J Nutr 2007;97:111–6.
[14] Ferris AM, Neubauer SH, Bendel RB, et al. Perinatal lactation protocol and outcome in mothers with and without insulin-dependent diabetes mellitus. Am J Clin Nutr 1993;58:43–8.
[15] Lammi-Keefe CJ, Jonas CR, Ferris AM, et al. Vitamin E in plasma and milk of lactating women with insulin dependent diabetes mellitus. J Pediatr Gastroenterol Nutr 1995;20:305–9.
[16] Neubauer SH, Ferris AM, Chanse CG, et al. Delayed lactogenesis in women with insulin-dependent diabetes mellitus. Am J Clin Nutr 1993;58:54–60.
[17] Ferris AM, Dalidowitz CK, Ingrdia DM, et al. Lactation outcome in insulin-dependent diabetic women. J Am Diet Assoc 1988;88:317–22.
[18] Kjos SL, Henry O, Lee RM, et al. The effect of lactation on glucose and lipid metabolism in women with recent gestational diabetes. Obstet Gynecol 1993;82:451–5.

[19] Preventing childhood obesity: health in balance. Washington, DC: Institute of Medicine of the National Academies; 2004. Available at: http://www.iom.edu/?id=22623. Accessed April 20, 2007.

[20] American Diabetes Association. Type 2 diabetes in children and adolescents. Diabetes Care 2000;23:381–9.

[21] Anonymous. The effect of intensive therapy of diabetes on the development and progression of long-term complications in insulin-dependent diabetes mellitus. The Diabetes Control and Complications Trial Research Group. N Engl J Med 1993;329:977–86.

[22] Anonymous. United Kingdom Prospective Diabetes Study 24: A 6-year, randomized, controlled trial comparing sulfonylurea, insulin and metformin therapy in patients with newly diagnosed type 2 diabetes that could not be controlled with diet therapy. Ann Intern Med 1998;128:165–75.

[23] American Diabetes Association. Implications of the United Kingdom Prospective Diabetes Study: reviews/commentaries/position statement: position statement. Diabetes Care 1998; 21:2180–4.

[24] UK Prospective Diabetes Study Group. Intensive blood-glucose control with sulphonylureas or insulin compared to conventional treatment and risk of complications in patients with type 2 diabetes (UKPDS 33). Lancet 1998;352:837–53.

[25] UK Prospective Diabetes Study Group. Intensive blood-glucose control with metformin on complications in overweight patients with type 2 diabetes (UKPDS 34). Lancet 1998;352: 854–65.

[26] Fuhrman K, Reiher H, Semmler K, et al. The effect of intensified conventional insulin therapy before and during pregnancy on the malformation rate in offspring of diabetic mothers. Exp Clin Endocrinol 1984;83:173.

[27] UK Prospective Diabetes Study Group. Tight blood pressure control and risk of macrovascular and microvascular complications in type 2 diabetes. (UKPDS 38). BMJ 1998;317: 703–13.

[28] Cooper WO, Hernandez-Diaz S, Arbogast PG, et al. Major congenital malformations after first-trimester exposure to ACE inhibitors. N Engl J Med 2006;354(23):2443–51.

[29] Kjos SL, Buchanan TA, Montoro M, et al. Serum lipids within thirty-six months of delivery in women with recent gestational diabetes mellitus. Diabetes 1991;40(Suppl 2): 142–6.

[30] Expert Panel on Detection, Evaluation, and Treatment of High Blood Cholesterol in Adults. Executive summary of Third Report of The National Cholesterol Education Program (NCEP) Expert Panel on detection, evaluation, and treatment of high blood cholesterol in adults (Adult Treatment Panel III). JAMA 2001;285:2486–97.

[31] Kim C, Newton KM, Knopp RH. Gestational diabetes and the incidence of type 2 diabetes. Diabetes Care 2002;25:1862–8.

[32] Schaefer-Graf UM, Buchanan TA, Xiang AH, et al. Clinical predictors for high risk for developing diabetes in the early puerperium in women with recent gestational diabetes. Am J Obstet Gynecol 2002;186(4):751–6.

[33] Buchanan TA, Xiang AH, Kjos SL, et al. Antepartum predictors of the development of type 2 diabetes in Latino women 11–26 months after pregnancies complicated by gestational diabetes. Diabetes 1999;48:2430–6.

[34] Lauenborg J, Hansen T, Jensen DM, et al. Increasing incidence of diabetes after gestational diabetes. Diabetes Care 2004;27(5):1194–9.

[35] Kjos SL, Peters RK, Xiang A, et al. Predicting future diabetes in Latino women with gestational diabetes: utility of early postpartum glucose tolerance testing. Diabetes 1995;44: 586–91.

[36] Kousta E, Lawrence NJ, Penny A, et al. Implications of new diagnostic criteria for abnormal glucose homeostasis in women with previous gestational diabetes. Diabetes Care 1999;22: 933–7.

[37] Pallardo LF, Herranz L, Martin-Vaquero P, et al. Impaired fasting glucose and impaired glucose tolerance in women with prior gestational diabetes are associated with different cardiovascular profiles. Diabetes Care 2003;26:2318–22.

[38] Metzger BE, Buchanan TA, Coustan DR, et al. Summary and recommendations of the Fifth International Workshop Conference on Gestational Diabetes Mellitus. Diabetes Care, in press.

[39] Damm P, Kuhl C, Bertelsen A, et al. Predictive factors for the development of diabetes in women with previous gestational diabetes mellitus. Am J Obstet Gynecol 1992;167: 607–16.

[40] Diabetes Prevention Program Research Group. Reduction in the incidence of type 2 diabetes with lifestyle intervention or metformin. N Engl J Med 2002;346:393–403.

[41] Tuomilehto J, Lindström J, Eriksson J, et al. Prevention of type 2 diabetes mellitus by changes in lifestyle among subjects with impaired glucose tolerance. N Engl J Med 2001; 344:1343–50.

[42] Chisson JL, Josse RG, Gomis R, et al, STOP-NIDDM Trial Research Group. JAMA 2003; 290:486–94.

[43] Torgerson JS, Hauptman J, Boldrin MN, et al. XENical in prevention of diabetes in obese subjects for the prevention of type 2 diabetes in obese patients. Diabetes Care 2004;27: 155–61.

[44] Buchanan TA, Xiang AH, Peters RK, et al. The TRIPOD Study: preservation of pancreatic B-cell function and prevention of type 2 diabetes by pharmacological treatment of insulin resistance in high-risk Hispanic women. Diabetes 2002;9:2796–803.

[45] American Diabetes Association. Nutrition recommendations and principles for people with diabetes mellitus. Diabetes Care 2006;29:2140–57.

[46] American Diabetes Association. Diabetes mellitus and exercise. Diabetes Care 2002;25: S64–9.

[47] Usui K, Yamanouchi K, Asai K, et al. The effect of low intensity bicycle exercise on insulin-induced glucose uptake in obese patients with type 2 diabetes. Diabetes Res Clin Pract 1998; 41:57–61.

[48] Giacca A, Groenewoud Y, Tsui E, et al. Glucose production, utilization and cycling in response to moderate exercise in obese subjects with type 2 diabetes and mild hyperglycemia. Diabetes 1998;47:1763–70.

[49] Halle M, Berg A, Garwers U, et al. Influence of 4 weeks' intervention by exercise and diet on low-density lipoprotein subfractions in obese men with type 2 diabetes. Metab Clin Exp 1999;48:641–4.

[50] Dunstan DW, Mori TA, Puddley IB, et al. A randomized, controlled study of the effects of aerobic exercise and dietary fish on coagulation and fibrinolytic factors in type 2 diabetics. Thromb Haemost 1999;81:367–72.

[51] Eriksson KF, Lindegarde F. No excess 12-year mortality in men with impaired glucose tolerance who participated in the Malmo Preventive Trial with diet and exercise. Diabetologia 1998;41:1010–6.

[52] Pan X-R, Li G-W, Hu Y-H, et al. Effects of diet and exercise in preventing NIDDM in people with impaired glucose tolerance: the Da Qing IGT and Diabetes Study. Diabetes Care 1997; 20:537–44.

[53] Gregory KD, Kjos SL, Peters RK. Cost of non-insulin-dependent diabetes in women with a history of gestational diabetes: Implications for prevention. Obstet Gynecol 1993;81: 782–6.

[54] Pettitt DJ, Baird HR, Aleck KA, et al. Excessive obesity in offspring of Pima Indian women with diabetes during pregnancy. N Engl J Med 1983;308:242–5.

[55] Pettitt DJ, Bennett PH, Knowler WC, et al. Gestational diabetes mellitus and impaired glucose tolerance during pregnancy: long-term effects on obesity and glucose tolerance in the offspring. Diabetes 1985;34(Suppl 2):119–22.

[56] Pettitt DJ, Knowler WC. Long-term effects of the intrauterine environment, birth weight, and breast-feeding on Pima Indians. Diabetes Care 1998;21(Suppl 2):B138–41.

[57] Silverman BL, Rizzo T, Green OC, et al. Long-term prospective evaluation of offspring of diabetic mothers. Diabetes 1991;40(Suppl2):121–5.

[58] Silverman BL, Rizzo TA, Cho NH, Metzger BE. Long-term effects of the intrauterine environment. Diabetes Care 1998;21(Suppl 2):B142–9.

[59] Helmrich SP, Ragland DR, Leung RW, et al. Physical activity and reduced occurrence of non-insulin dependent diabetes. N Engl J Med 1991;325:147–52.

[60] Manson JE, Rimm EB, Stampfer MJ, et al. Physical activity and incidence of non-insulin-dependent diabetes mellitus in women. Lancet 1991;338:774–8.

[61] US Department of Health and Human Services. Physical Activity and Health: A Report of the Surgeon General. Centers for Disease Control and Prevention, National Center for Chronic Disease Prevention and Health Promotion. Washington, DC: US Government Printing Office; 1996.

[62] Campbel OM, Gray RH. Characteristics and determinants of postpartum ovarian function in women in the United States. Am J Obstet Gynecol 1993;169:55–60.

[63] Perez A, Labbok MH, Queenan JT. Clinical study of the lactational amenorrhoea method for family planning. Lancet 1992;339:968–70.

[64] Kennedy KI, Rivera R, McNeilly AS. Consensus statement on the use of breastfeeding as a family planning method. Contraception 1989;39:477–96.

[65] Labbok M, Perez A, Valdes V, et al. The lactational Amenorrhea Method (LAM): a postpartum introductory family planning method with policy and program implications. Adv Contraception 1994;10:93–109.

[66] World Health Organization (WHO). Medical Eligibility Criteria for Contraceptive Use, 3rd edition. 2004. Geneva, Switzerland. 2004. (http://www.who.int/reproductive-health/publications/mec/index.htm).

[67] Truit ST, Fraser AB, Grimes DA, et al. Combined hormonal versus nonhormonal versus progestin-only contraception in lactation. Chochrane Syst Rev 2003;(2):CDC003988.

[68] World Health Organization (WHO). Selected Practice Recommendations for Contraceptive Use. Geneva: Switzerland; 2002.

[69] Faculty of Family Planning and Reproductive Health Care Clinical Effectiveness Unit. Family Planning and Reproductive Health Care Guidance (July 2004). Contraceptive choices for breastfeeding women. Journal of Family Planning and Reproductive Health Care 2004;30:181–9.

[70] ACOG Educational Bulletin No 258, Breastfeeding: maternal and infant aspects. American College of Obstetricians and Gynecologists 2004 Compendium of Selected Publications, Washington DC, 2004.

[71] Mills JL, Baker L, Goldman AS. Malformations in infants of diabetic mothers occur before the seventh gestational week. Diabetes 1979;28:292–3.

[72] Towner D, Kjos SL, Leung B, et al. Congenital malformations in pregnancies complicated by NIDDM. Diabetes Care 1995;18:1446–51.

[73] Schaefer UM, Songster G, Xiang A, et al. Congenital malformations in offspring of women with hyperglycemia first detected during pregnancy. Am J Obstet Gynecol 1997;177:1165–71.

[74] Radberg T, Gustafson A, Skryten A, et al. Oral contraception in diabetic women. Diabetes control, serum and high-density lipoprotein lipids during low-dose progestogen, combined oestrogen/progestogen and non-hormonal contraception. Acta Endocrinol 1981;98:246–51.

[75] Skouby SO, Jensen BM, Kuhl C, et al. Hormonal contraception in diabetic women: acceptability and influence on diabetes control and ovarian function of a nonalkylated estrogen/progestogen compound. Contraception 1985;32:23–31.

[76] Peterson KR, Skouby SO, Sidelmann J, et al. Effects of contraceptive steroids on cardiovascular risk factors in women with insulin-dependent diabetes mellitus. Am J Obstet Gynecol 1994;171:400–5.

[77] Petersen KR, Skouby SO, Sidelmann J, et al. Assessment of endothelial function during oral contraception in women with insulin -dependent diabetes mellitus. Metabol Clinical Exper 1994;43:1379–83.
[78] Klein BEK, Moss SE, Klein R. Oral contraceptives in women with diabetes. Diabetes Care 1990;13:895–8.
[79] Garg SK, Chase HP, Marshal G, et al. Oral contraceptives and renal and retinal complications in young women with insulin- dependent diabetes mellitus. JAMA 1994;271:1099–102.
[80] Skouby SO, Kuhl C, Molsted-Pedersen L, et al. Triphasic oral contraception: Metabolic effects in normal women and those with previous gestational diabetes. Am J Obstet Gyncol 1985;153:495–500.
[81] Skouby SO, Anderson O, Saurbrey N, et al. Oral contraception and insulin sensitivity: in vivo assessment in normal women and women with previous gestational diabetes. J Clin Endocrinol Metab 1987;64:519–23.
[82] Kjos SL, Shoupe D, Douyan S, et al. Effect of low-dose oral contraceptives on carbohydrate and lipid metabolism in women with recent gestational diabetes: results of a controlled, randomized, prospective study. Am J Obstet Gynecol 1990;163:1822–7.
[83] Kjos SL, Peters RK, Xiang A, et al. Contraception and the risk of type 2 diabetes mellitus in Latina women with prior gestational diabetes mellitus. JAMA 1998;280:533–8.
[84] Xiang AH, Kawakubo M, Kjos SL, et al. Long-acting injectable progestin contraception and risk of type 2 diabetes in Latino women with prior gestational diabetes mellitus. Diabetes Care 2006;29:613–7.
[85] Kjos SL. Contraception in diabetic women. Obstet Gynecol Clin N Am 1996;23:243–58.
[86] Farley TMM, Rosenberg MJ, Rowe PJ, et al. Intrauterine devices and pelvic inflammatory disease: an international perspective. Lancet 1992;339:785–8.
[87] Skouby SO, Molsted-Pedersen A. Consequences of intrauterine contraception in diabetic women. Fert Steril 1984;42:568–72.
[88] Kimmerle R, Weiss R, Berger M, et al. Effectiveness, safety and acceptability of a copper intrauterine device (CU Safe 300) in type I diabetic women. Diabetes Care 1993;16:1227–30.
[89] Kjos SL, Ballagh SA, La Cour M, et al. The copper T380A intrauterine device in women with type II diabetes mellitus. Obstet Gynecol 1994;84:1006–9.

**ELSEVIER
SAUNDERS**

Obstet Gynecol Clin N Am
34 (2007) 351–356

**OBSTETRICS AND
GYNECOLOGY
CLINICS
OF NORTH AMERICA**

# Index

*Note:* Page numbers of article titles are in **boldface** type.

## A

Acidosis, fetal, and stillbirth, 300

Adaptive immune system, in gestational diabetes mellitus, 216, 218–219

Adiponectin, and insulin resistance, in gestational diabetes mellitus, 218

Adipose tissue development, in offspring of diabetic mothers, animal models of, 207

Adipose tissue, in gestational diabetes mellitus, 217

Alpha-glucosidase inhibitors, for gestational diabetes mellitus, 268–269

Amenorrhea, lactation, as birth control method, 342–343

Antepartum fetal surveillance, in gestational diabetes mellitus, to prevent stillbirth, 302–304

Anti-hyperglycemic agents, oral. *See* Oral anti-hyperglycemic agents.

Anti-inflammatory response, decreased, in gestational diabetes mellitus, 219

Appetite regulating systems, exposure of, to leptin, 206

Appetite regulation, in offspring, gestational diabetes mellitus and, animal models of, 205–206

Artificial pancreas, for gestational diabetes mellitus, 250

## B

B10Asp insulin, for gestational diabetes mellitus, 285

Beta-cell dysfunction, in gestational diabetes mellitus, 215

Biguanides, for gestational diabetes mellitus. *See* Oral anti-hyperglycemic agents.

Biophysical profile, in antepartum surveillance, to prevent stillbirth, 303

Biparietal diameter, in detection of macrosomia, 319

Blood pressure control, to prevent cardiovascular complications, of gestational diabetes mellitus, 339

Breastfeeding
as birth control method, 342–343
gestational diabetes mellitus and, 337

## C

Carbohydrate intolerance, reduction of, in offspring of diabetic mothers, 337–338

Cardiovascular function, in offspring, gestational diabetes mellitus and, animal models of, 208

Cesarean section, in gestational diabetes mellitus, 328–329

Cheek-to-cheek diameter, in detection of macrosomia, 319

Childhood obesity, reduction of, in offspring of diabetic mothers, 337–338

Combined oral contraceptives, postpartum, gestational diabetes mellitus and, 343–344

Congenital malformations, gestational diabetes mellitus and, 174, 226–229, 326–327
insulin analogues and, 279
oral anti-hyperglycemic agents and, 265–266
prevention of, 227–229

Contraception, postpartum. *See* Gestational diabetes mellitus, postpartum care for.

Coronary heart disease, with gestational diabetes mellitus, periconceptional care for, 232–233, 235

reduction of later childhood
obesity in newborn,
337–338
reduction of risk for diabetes or
complications, 338–342
blood pressure control
in, 339
fasting plasma glucose
in, 340
for women with prior
gestational diabetes,
339–341
for women with type 1 and
2 diabetes, 338–339
lifestyle intervention in,
341–342
normalizing serum lipid
levels in, 339
oral glucose tolerance test
in, 340
self-monitoring of blood
glucose in, 338–339
reproductive health and
contraception in, 342–344
combined oral
contraceptives in,
343–344
intrauterine devices in, 344
lactation amenorrhea
method in, 342–343
oral contraceptives in,
343–344
progestin-only oral
contraceptives in,
343–344
return of ovulation in, 342
prevalence of, **173–199**
difficulties in comparing,
192–193
early life exposures and, 174
ethnicity in, 174, 175, 178, 185,
189, 192–193
global, 173
public health impact of,
193–194
studies on, 175–177
diagnostic criteria in, 176
hospital-based studies, 179,
185
literature searches in, 175
population-based studies,
177–179
results of, 177–189
screening and definitions in,
175–176
trends in, 185, 189

Glucose levels, postpartum management of,
in gestational diabetes mellitus,
335–337, 338–339

Glucose metabolism, in pregnancy,
213–214

Glucose monitoring, in gestational diabetes
mellitus, **241–253**
artificial pancreas in, 250
from glucosuria to continuous
monitoring, 241–247
for treatment adjustment, 247
for treatment assessment, 246
glycosylated hemoglobin and
protein, 242
in insulin-treated women, 246
postprandial glycemic profile,
245–246
self-monitoring, 242–243
technology for, 243–244
versus nondiabetic pregnancy,
244–245
insulin pump in, 247–249
disadvantages and side effects
of, 248
versus conventional therapy, 249

Glyburide, for gestational diabetes mellitus,
260–263

Glycemic control
in nonpregnancy, 247–248
intrapartum/peripartum, and labor
and delivery, 329–330

Glycemic profile
in nondiabetic pregnancy, 244–245
postprandial, in gestational diabetes
mellitus, 245–246

Glycosylated fructosamine, to measure
glycemic level, in gestational diabetes
mellitus, 242

Glycosylated hemoglobin, to measure
glycemic level, in gestational diabetes
mellitus, 242

Glycosylated protein, to measure glycemic
level, in gestational diabetes mellitus,
242

## H

Hemoglobin A1c levels, in gestational
diabetes mellitus, and stillbirth, 302

Hormonal contraception, postpartum,
gestational diabetes mellitus and,
343–344

Hypertension, in gestational
diabetes mellitus
and diabetic retinopathy, 232
and labor and delivery,
325–326

# Moving?

## Make sure your subscription moves with you!

To notify us of your new address, find your **Clinics Account Number** (located on your mailing label above your name), and contact customer service at:

E-mail: elspcs@elsevier.com

800-654-2452 (subscribers in the U.S. & Canada)
407-345-4000 (subscribers outside of the U.S. & Canada)

Fax number: 407-363-9661

**Elsevier Periodicals Customer Service**
6277 Sea Harbor Drive
Orlando, FL  32887-4800

*To ensure uninterrupted delivery of your subscription, please notify us at least 4 weeks in advance of move.